PRAISE FOR
MEAL PREP YOUR WAY TO WEIGHT LOSS

"Nikki is an authority on what to eat, and she breaks it down in an easy-to-understand way that will set you up for success. Meal prepping is one of the keys to success, and her book shows you all the steps needed to master this, master your diet, and see the results you want."

—Jason Wachob, founder and CEO of mindbodygreen and author of *Wellth*

"For optimal mental performance, there are certain non-negotiables—top of the list is eating the right brain foods consistently. Nikki Sharp makes it easy, rewarding, and fun in her new book. Her meal-prepping process is a simple and powerful way to nourish your mind. Bottom line, devour this book because the foods we eat matter, especially to our gray matter."

—Jim Kwik, celebrity memory coach and host of the *Kwik Brain* podcast

"If you want to succeed at anything in life, you have to be prepared. If you truly want to eat healthy, meal prepping is the only way. You cannot leave your food options to chance. I've never been more inspired to meal prep in my life. Thank you, Nikki, for writing such a beautiful book with so many delicious and easy meal prep options."

—Sarah DeAnna, model and author of *Supermodel YOU*

"In *Meal Prep Your Way to Weight Loss,* Nikki Sharp rightfully places diet as the centerpiece of a healthy lifestyle. She makes taking the first step on the road to health an easy one, which anyone who leads a busy life will surely value. This book is a must-read if you want to change habits, learn how to meal prep, and stop dieting once and for all!"

—Max Lugavere, author of *Genius Foods*

"Nikki is an inspiration to her friends and followers, and she's just like us. I love that her new book explores real-life problems, avoids dieting, and instead gives strategic meal-prep advice to avoid emotional eating and enable us to eat clean every week!"

—Kelly LeVeque, celebrity nutritionist and author of *Body Love*

"As a professional chef, I am thrilled to see Nikki Sharp creating an entire book built around what we call *mis en place*. Her recipes are always vibrant and colorful, while also being nutritious and delicious. In her new book, she has taken the concept of recipes and healthy eating to a new level by focusing on what home cooks need most: guidance on how to organize the food prep for success."
—Matthew Kenney, chef, entrepreneur, and author of *PLANTLAB*

"In her new book, Nikki breaks down meal prep so that anyone can succeed—whether they've tried it before or not. Not to mention, the recipes are beautiful and delicious."
—Jordan Younger, host of the *Soul on Fire* podcast and founder of *The Balanced Blonde*

"A must-read! If you've been stuck in the diet cycle, Nikki's new book will completely change that. It teaches you everything you need to know about emotional eating, how to stop it, and how powerful meal prep is!"
—Tara Mackey, author of *WILD Habits*

"Eating well doesn't happen by accident! Planning is the first step in any worthy endeavor, and Nikki Sharp has made it so easy for you to follow in her healthy footsteps. Get the skinny on organizing your meals!"
—Lorie Marrero, *Wall Street Journal* bestselling author of *The Clutter Diet*

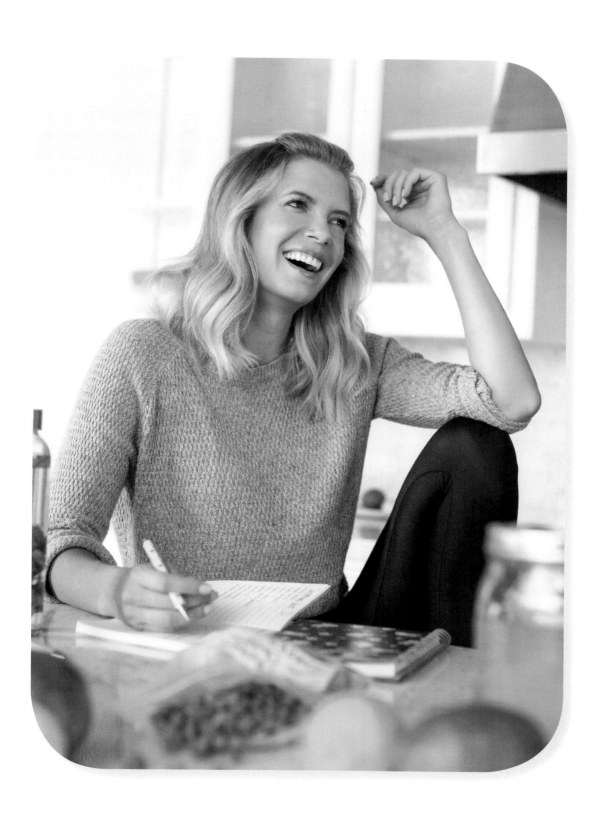

BY NIKKI SHARP

Meal Prep Your Way to Weight Loss
The 5-Day Real Food Detox

Meal Prep Your Way to Weight Loss

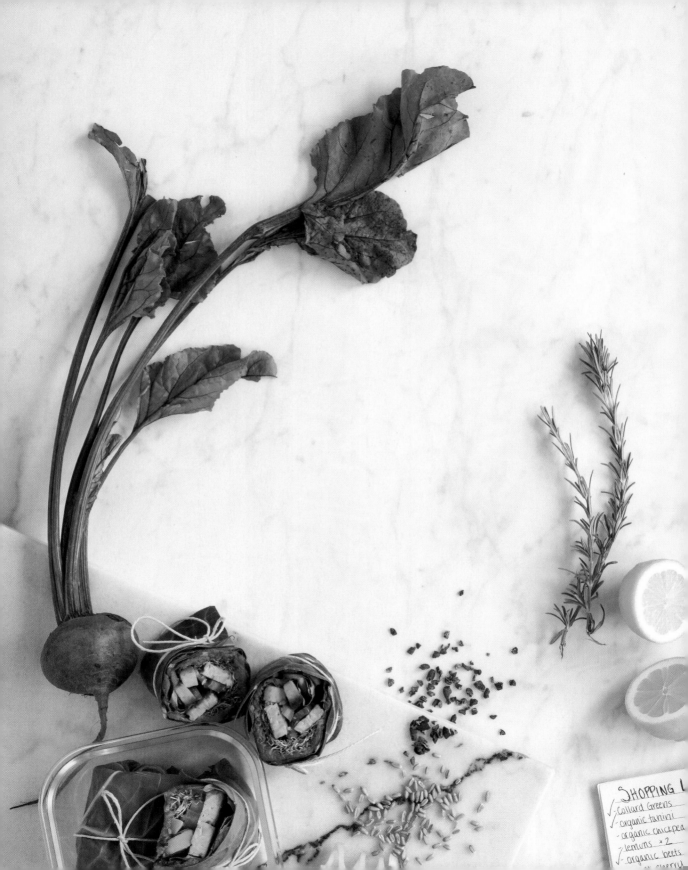

SHOPPING L
✓ Collard Greens
✓ organic tahini
- organic chickpea
✓ lemons × 2
✓ organic beets

Meal Prep Your Way to Weight Loss

28 Days to a Fitter, Healthier You

NIKKI SHARP

BALLANTINE BOOKS

NEW YORK

Meal Prep Your Way to Weight Loss proposes a program of dietary and nutrition recommendations for the reader to follow. No book, however, can replace the diagnostic and medical expertise of a qualified physician. Please consult your doctor (and, if you are pregnant, your ob/gyn) before making sustained or extensive changes in your diet, particularly if you suffer from any diagnosed medical condition or have any symptoms that may require treatment.

As of the time of initial publication, the URLs displayed in this book link or refer to existing websites on the Internet. Penguin Random House LLC is not responsible for, and should not be deemed to endorse or recommend, any website other than its own or any content available on the Internet (including without limitation at any website, blog page, information page) that is not created by Penguin Random House.

A Ballantine Books Trade Paperback Original

Published in the United States by Ballantine Books, an imprint of Random House, a division of Penguin Random House LLC, New York.

BALLANTINE and the HOUSE colophon are registered trademarks of Penguin Random House LLC.

Photos on pages *x* and *xii* are courtesy of the author.
All remaining photos are © Pam McLean
Kitchen frame illustration on pages 3, 53, 123, 132–35, 155–59, 183–88, and 211–16 © istock/naeinbil
Meal clock illustration on pages 132, 155, 183, and 211 © istock/zak00

LIBRARY OF CONGRESS CATALOGING-IN-PUBLICATION DATA
Names: Sharp, Nikki, author.
Title: Meal prep your way to weight loss : 28 days to a fitter, healthier you / Nikki Sharp.
Description: New York : Ballantine Books, [2018]
Identifiers: LCCN 2018002191 | ISBN 9781101886946 (paperback) | ISBN 9781101886953 (ebook)
Subjects: LCSH: Weight loss. | Nutrition. | Health. | Reducing diets—Recipes. | BISAC: COOKING / Health & Healing / General. | HEALTH & FITNESS / Diets. | HEALTH & FITNESS / Weight Loss.
Classification: LCC RM222.2 .S483 2018 | DDC 641.5/637—dc23
LC record available at https://lccn.loc.gov/2018002191

Printed in the United States of America on acid-free paper

randomhousebooks.com

10 9 8 7 6 5 4 3 2 1

Food stylist: John Anthony Galang

Book design by Diane Hobbing

Chocolate comes from cocoa, which is a tree. That makes it a plant. Chocolate is salad.

—ANONYMOUS

This book is dedicated to everyone who wants to live a happy and healthy life . . . while still eating chocolate!

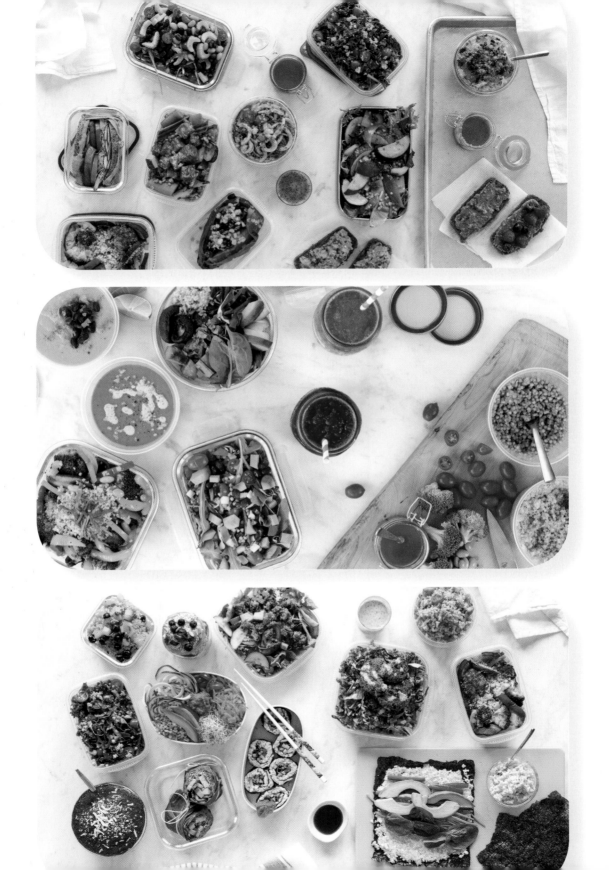

CONTENTS

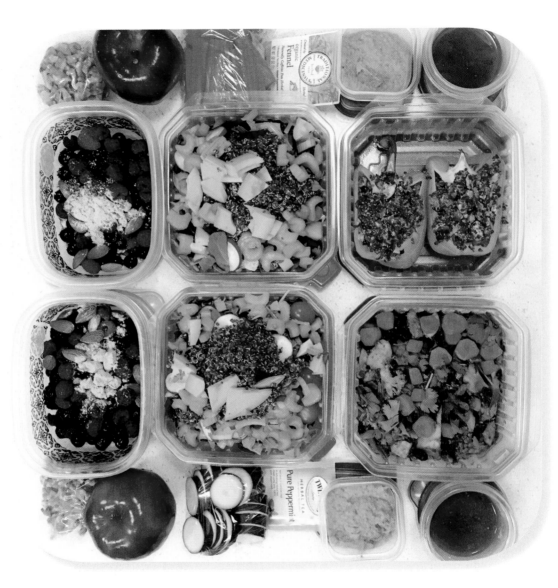

INTRODUCTION

After my first book, *The 5-Day Real Food Detox,* was published, I was excited about writing a second book. The question was what *kind* of book. I didn't just want to write a cookbook, because even with a hundred recipes at your fingers in this book, cooking and eating healthy can be daunting. Don't get me wrong—I love creating recipes and showcasing "sexy," healthy food. I love teaching people how to make delicious meals, and I love showing people how healthy food tastes better than anything they could ever imagine.

But was that what my readers needed?

I knew deep down that shifting out of detox mode and back into everyday eating could easily be a recipe for disaster. Without a routine, shopping and cooking can be time-consuming, expensive, and confusing. I realized then that I wanted to write something to eliminate the slippery slope that can lead to making unhealthy food choices.

Nutrition is definitely confusing, even to me, and so while I wholeheartedly believe in eating healthier, more nutrient-dense whole foods, I didn't want to write a book that was simply about following the latest health trends. I needed to write something that would truly inspire people to make positive changes in their lives, while helping them to navigate all the conflicting information out there about health and wellness. But what exactly would that look like?

Let me back up a moment. Over the years, I've had many celebrities do my 5-Day Real Food Detox. Once, a celeb wanted to follow my plan before appearing on a big awards show. I prepped the entire detox for him to save time and make sure he stuck with the program in order to see the results he wanted before the red carpet. Prior to delivering it to him on the set, I sent him a photo of his food, all laid out. I posted it on my Instagram account, and he posted it on his.

The next day, I awoke to mass emails, texts, and messages, saying that a picture of me, along with this photo, had landed on the front page of the *Daily Mail* website.

What will YOU have for lunch today? The incredibly organized (or smug) 'meal queens' who spend Sundays making a week's worth of healthy food guaranteed to make co-workers green with envy

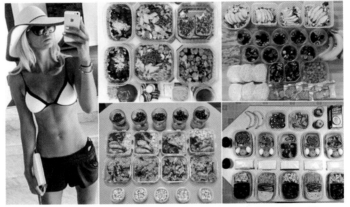

Everyone knows that smug co-worker who arrives to the office with a perfectly packed healthy lunch. Now, meal-prepping has become an Instagram movement. From fitness gurus and would-be health nuts to time poor mums and young working women, meal prepping is popping up on everyone's social media feeds. It's a way to save time during the week, plan your meals, and ensure you're eating well and stick to your health plan. And Instagram provides plenty of healthy eating inspiration in the form of the hashtags #mealprep and #mealprepdaily which boast tens of thousands of photos. Left: American 'wellness expert and health coach' Nikki Sharp is a fan of meal planning, posting quite a few snaps on Instagram of her prepped food.

💬 **597** comments   ▶️ **1 video**   ⤴ **950 shares**

It talked about meal prepping and dubbed me the "Meal Prep Queen of Instagram." That very same day, I had various other magazines and online publications, such as *Business Insider,* reach out to me to showcase this new "trend." I did interviews on the topic and created videos for it. After the quick media blitz died down, I went on with my life and did the work of promoting my first book.

Later in the summer, while I was thinking about writing my second book, I remembered this story, and I had that aha moment: meal prep!

I needed to write about meal prepping—a health trend that has become increasingly popular but still isn't something that most people know how to do. I realized that by teaching people how to meal prep, I could help them lose weight—and achieve other health goals they have, which leads to living happier and healthier lives. While there is still a lot of back-and-forth as to what diet is healthiest, no one can deny that meal prepping your food, bringing your own lunches to work, and having ready-to-eat homemade meals in the fridge at home is effective for so many various reasons.

And so began *Meal Prep Your Way to Weight Loss.*

Did I invent meal prepping? No. But I've done it affordably and sustainably for years. Now I want to show you how to do it too, all while saving money and eating food that you'll love even as you are still losing weight. My method is so incredibly simple—and it will revolutionize the way you go about planning and cooking your meals.

I know what you're thinking, because I've heard it before: "Why should I listen to her? She has a great body and doesn't have to worry about weight."

Au contraire, my friend. I have gone through ups and downs like everyone else.

Growing up, I tried every single diet you can imagine. I mean seriously—name it, and I tried it. This was the age of Atkins, South Beach, cabbage soup dieting, and so many more. Why did I do them all? Because I thought I needed to lose weight, which sadly had nothing to do with my health. I then began modeling and stopped the dieting—because I just stopped eating entirely. It was not a healthy way to live, and it took its toll. I was fatigued and anxious. I had an incredibly poor body image. I suffered from insomnia and depression, and I had terrible skin.

I was also clueless about what good nutrition really meant. For example, I believed that drinking milk every day was okay. It's not, since milk can be allergenic, is high in the sugar lactose, and often is loaded with hormones and toxins.* I thought that the sauces used in vegetable stir-fries were harmless. Not at all: they are full of chemicals, salt, and preservatives. I thought that fruit smoothies were the healthiest choices on the planet. Now I know better: too much fruit can spike blood sugar and lead to hunger pangs later on, not to mention weight gain.

As for weight loss? I tried to practically starve myself skinny. I subsisted on hard-boiled eggs, lettuce, and diet soda. Then I binged for years in retaliation.

Therein lies the problem. When we diet or skip meals, we think that we are doing something good for ourselves. But we aren't. We feel restricted and lose control, which in turn can lead to bingeing.

For these reasons, I'm not a big proponent of restrictive diet plans. They focus too much on what to eliminate from your diet, rather than how to eat for health and success (and trust me, I know this from trying so many diets!). Dieting traps you in a negative state of mind, whereas eating for health allows you to think about food in a positive way and helps you feel happy about your life and your choices.

So, after all my dieting, swinging back and forth from starving to bingeing and feeling terrible about myself, I'd had enough. My body finally screamed out: *"Feed me!"*

Slowly, I began to learn about the right way to feed my body. I also began to focus on incorporating wholesome practices into my life: a colorful, plant-based diet, yoga, meditation, journaling, and more. I concentrated on what I wanted to add to my life, rather than on what I should eliminate. The more I ate healthy foods and followed this new lifestyle, the happier I felt about my body and my life. Physical and emotional problems started to disappear. The more I learned, though, the more I realized that healthy foods needed to be in my fridge, ready to eat; otherwise, I wouldn't touch them. That's when meal prepping became central to my life.

You and I both know that foods like Brussels sprouts are good for us. But there's no way we're coming home from a long day and cooking them. Sure, it's in our best interest to do so, but we all lead busy lives and

* No wonder I had ongoing terrible acne since I was 11!

we have to be realistic. Instead, when we are busy, we grab the most convenient foods to eat, which in almost all cases are loaded with salt, sugar, chemicals, and other junk that is not giving us what our bodies need. But if those Brussels sprouts and other healthy foods are prepped and cooked ahead of time, we can just reheat them quickly and enjoy.

So I began to make sure not only that my fridge was stocked with delicious healthy foods but also that these foods were prepared and ready to eat. The more I meal prepped, the better my results.

Success came from having salad ingredients precut and easy to throw together, and quinoa, beans, lentils, shredded chicken, hard-boiled eggs, and other foods tucked into containers in my fridge. There's more: portion sizes of hummus and veggies, nuts, and fruit salads that I could grab and go, and water in bottles that had lemon and lime slices in them. Nothing I prepped was complicated or too time-consuming. I made simple yet incredibly healthy and delicious meals.

I meal prepped every week, and I got better and better at it. Meal prepping became second nature to me, and soon I could fix an entire week's worth of food in just a few hours. Along the way, I discovered my own little tricks of the trade that no one else was doing. Meal prepping was the answer to controlling my weight, feeling great about my body, and having health benefits such as increased energy, clearer skin, and a feeling of being in control of my food. It stopped the bingeing, and I felt excited about each meal I had prepped.

It was only a matter of time before my social media followers wanted to know more about how to eat healthy, create delicious and easy-to-follow meal plans, and save money while doing so. Those who had followed my 5-Day Real Food Detox desired to know more about what to do after the five days were over. And so this book was born: a guide to meal prepping, with a 28-day weight-loss and weight-control plan.

In the following pages, you'll learn three important things. First, you'll learn my life-changing, health-altering meal prep system. Second, you'll discover "super meals" and how they infuse ultra-nutrition into every bite of food. And finally, you'll be given my 28-day weight-loss plan, in which you meal prep your foods—breakfast, lunch, dinner, and snacks—each week, with ease. There's an added bonus: nearly 100 brand-new recipes!

And most important, you'll become a meal prep master, with all its benefits:

- Steady, satisfying weight loss—up to 5 pounds each week that you will keep off.
- Mastery of the simple skills of meal prepping.
- Automatic portion control—no counting calories, fat grams, carbohydrates, or any of that nonsense.
- Recipes for breakfast, lunch, dinner, and snacks so delicious you won't even know you're on a weight-loss plan.
- Control over what you put in your body.
- Meals that heal and renew your body, thanks to miracle nutrients rich in antioxidants and disease-fighting plant chemicals.
- An escape from emotional eating and bingeing.
- Stress-free cooking and eating—and an overall stress-free lifestyle.
- More time and money to enjoy your life.
- Attainment of the weight, energy, and health you so want and deserve.

By picking up this book and reading it, you are on your way to success. Every new bit of information you learn will help you create lasting habits. The meals in the book will nourish your body, and I promise you won't miss your old ways. Think of this book and its plan not as another diet, but as a new way of life.

Welcome to my meal prep weight-loss solution!

Meal Prep Your Way to Weight Loss

Part One

Lose Weight,
Meal by Meal

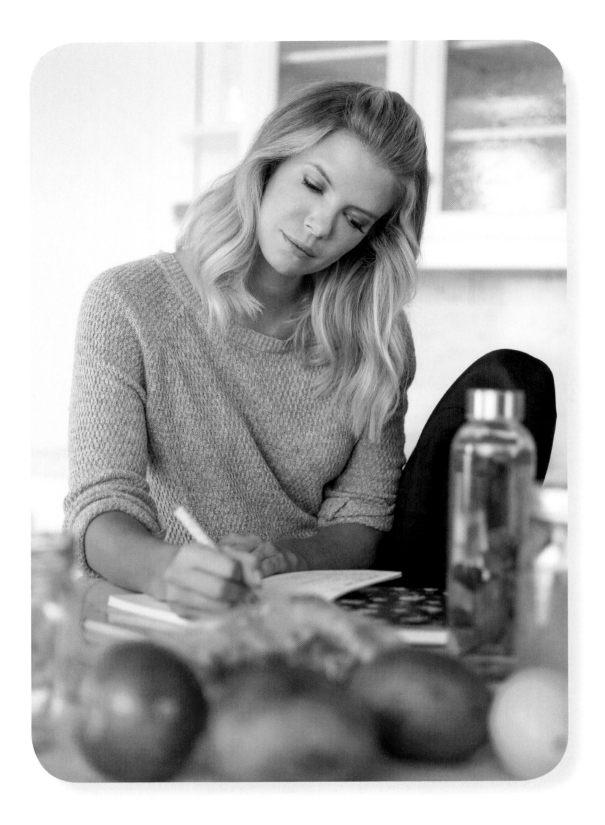

CHAPTER 1

Real "Fast Food" for *Real* Weight Loss

Imagine how you'd feel if you were at your dream weight—healthier, more energetic, and happier than you've ever been. Imagine if you could get there hassle-free, without spending countless hours in the kitchen or thinking obsessively about what you're going to eat or how much of it you should eat. Picture a new way of eating that won't have you spending your days at the gym. Doesn't this sound like an ideal way to lose weight and get healthy? Now ask yourself, "What's stopping me?"

When I coach my clients, I find that they want to lose weight but can't find the time to cook. They detest boring, bland diet food. They hate obsessing over calories, carbs, and fat. Nor do they want to have to be on a mundane diet while all their friends eat whatever they want. They want to eat delicious food, spend minimal time preparing it, and watch those extra pounds fall off naturally.

Does any of this sound familiar? If so, then you're not alone. Not by a long shot. Getting in shape and staying healthy in today's world can definitely be challenging. Trust me when I say, been there, done that!

It took me a long time to become a health and wellness expert, and I experienced a lot of ups and downs in the process. As I described earlier, I was very unhealthy while I was modeling. Eventually I left the fashion industry and its pressures, but I still swung back and forth: I'd starve myself and overexercise, then I'd eat everything in sight, gain weight, and feel so bad about myself that I didn't want to exercise at all. Soon I couldn't sleep, so I relied on sleeping pills for the next five years. I fell into a dark place and didn't think there was any way out. It wasn't until I let go of the intense pressure I put on myself to be "perfect" that I began to get better.

Still, as I began my road back to health, I had no idea which path I should take. And it's no wonder: there are so many diets, fitness trends, and health products out there, and they all point in different—often opposite—directions. I was confused by all the information out there. Should I be paleo, vegan, or just raw before 4:00 PM? Should I go low-carb or high-carb? Or should I be focused on cleansing and fasting? Seriously, what was best? Should I treat breakfast as the most important meal of the day or skip it? Should I drink bulletproof-style coffee or swear off caffeine altogether?

I get questions like these all the time. Clients tell me they're scared of not eating enough animal protein, and yet they can't seem to understand why their digestion is terrible after eating meat at every meal. People are curious, and hungry for the right nutritional information—which is great. But with more information out there than ever before, there's also more room for confusion.

In this book, I make nutrition, dieting, and health easy to understand and effective for you. It all boils down to three simple secrets that will change your body and your life right now.

Secret #1: Weekly Meal Prep

During the week, after a long day of health and nutrition coaching, the last thing I want to worry about is making food. If there isn't something awaiting me in my fridge, ready to be heated and devoured, I know I'm in trouble. I might grab something less healthy or go out to eat or reach for something convenient that is just not good for my body.

I bet you've been in the same boat. In an online questionnaire administered by the Heart and Stroke Foundation of Canada in 2011 and reported on www.cbc.ca, 41 percent of respondents said healthy meals are too much trouble to prepare. Too much trouble? *Cha-ching!* That's music to the ears of every fast-food joint on the planet. They've convinced us that we have better things to do with our time than cook, when in reality, planning healthy meals and cooking for ourselves is probably the single best thing we can do for our weight and health, not to mention our bank account.

So just think . . . you open your fridge and there's a full week of healthy, delicious food that's prepped, neatly portioned, and ready to eat. Wouldn't that make sticking to your diet and achieving fat loss a lot easier? It would also reduce a lot of the health issues you or people you know might be facing.

Behold: the power of meal prep. In essence, it involves cooking up several meals ahead of time and packaging them in individual, portion-sized containers so they're ready to eat and enjoy.

Making all your food for the week in advance keeps you on track with healthy, convenient eating, week to week. The key to success is planning out all of your meals on the weekend—for most people, Sunday works well—then doing the shopping and the prep on the same day. You can also split your prep into two days, with Wednesday as your second meal prep day, so the prep isn't quite as labor intensive. If you're worried about food not being as fresh, then splitting your week into two is a great option.

Whatever day you choose to do your meal prep, the preparation itself will take only two to three hours. Compare that to spending one to two hours each day cooking—seven to fourteen hours a week! Meal prepping is a huge time-saver—and more than that, it will help you control your portion sizes, stop you from obsessing over what to eat, save you money on groceries, help you to achieve faster and easier weight loss, and other health goals. Meal prep is quite miraculous in everything it brings to the table—literally.

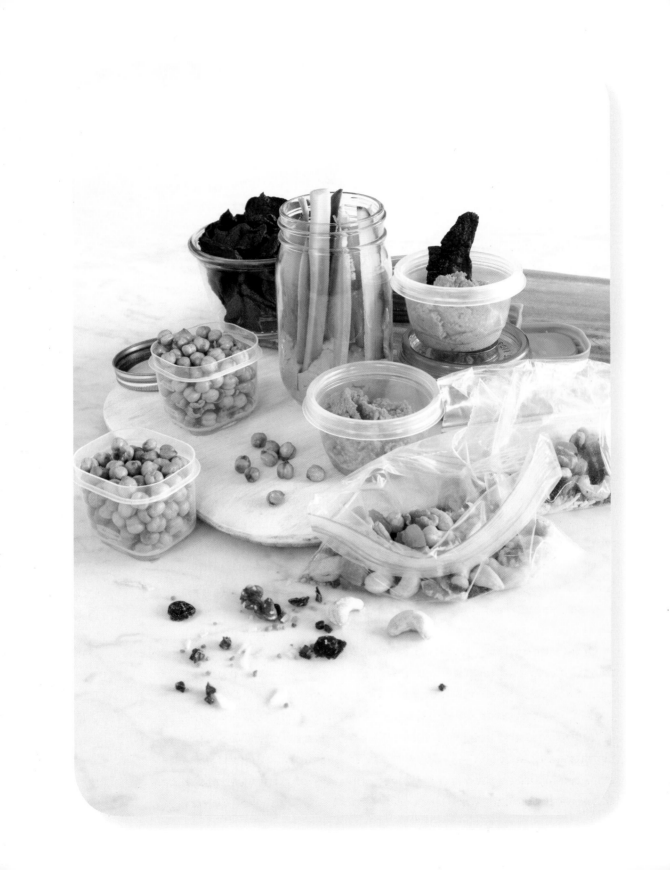

Secret #2: Plants!

So, what exactly are you going to be prepping? Mostly plant-based meals. I'm talking about vegetables, grains, fruits, and nuts. Yes, this is Secret #2 for keeping your weight down naturally and living a long and healthy life.

Here's some powerful evidence: vegetarian and vegan diets (both are plant based) that *skipped counting calories* produced greater weight loss over two months and kept the weight off at six months, compared to diets that included meat, according to a randomized, controlled study conducted at the Arnold School of Public Health at the University of South Carolina in Columbia.

The study was the first to directly compare the effects of five diets: vegan, vegetarian, pesco-vegetarian, semi-vegetarian, and omnivorous. All five diets focused on low-fat, low-glycemic-index foods (again, no calorie counting!). What's more, all five stressed eating foods that were as unprocessed as possible.

After just two months, participants eating the plant-based diets had lost an average of 8 to 10 pounds, while those eating meat lost an average of 5 pounds. At six months, the vegans had shed about 7 percent of their weight, the semi-vegetarian group had dropped about 4 percent of their weight, the pesco-vegetarian group had lost about 3 percent, and the meat group was also down about 3 percent.

So all groups lost a significant amount of weight without having to count calories, but the weight loss was highest in the vegan group. There was also much less intake of saturated fat and cholesterol in the vegan group.

Once I started prepping and eating clean, organic, and largely plant foods, I felt better mentally and emotionally. I felt less stressed, anxious, and depressed. I even started sleeping better.

Okay, so it worked for me. But can it work for you? Yes, I believe so.

In 2015, a paper in the journal *Nutritional Neuroscience* observed that vegans experienced less stress, anxiety, and depression than people who ate a mostly meat-based diet. The researchers noted that the "reduction of animal food intake may have mood benefits." Like me, you're probably wondering why that is. No explanation or evaluation was given, but I think it has to do with a number of known factors that affect our brains. One factor is that plant-based diets are extremely high in brain-friendly vitamins, like folate and B_6, and beneficial fats. Plant-based diets also steer you away from bad fats that tend to harm mood and mental performance while increasing your intake of essential fatty acids from good fats, such as flaxseeds, walnuts, and olive oil.

Another reason you'll feel better on a plant-based diet is that you're not ingesting the hormones found in most meat products. We take on the energy of the things we eat, and when animals are not raised in a loving environment, their stress hormones accumulate in their bodies—and those hormones wind up in our favorite steak. This is why it's so important to purchase local and organic products as often as possible. Yes, organic can be more expensive (more later on combatting priciness by buying in bulk!), but it's worth it. Not only will the food taste better, but you will feel better.

The food we eat is vitally important: it affects everything from our emotional health to our skin health, from our energy levels to our brain function. Not only is eating lots of fruits and vegetables an ideal way to feel great and shed pounds, but mounting research shows that plants are packed with powerful compounds called phytochemicals that boost your immunity, protect against disease, and fight fat.

To get these benefits, we must eat a wide variety of colorful foods. The more colorful a fruit or veggie, the more health-building nutrients it contains. Red foods, such as tomatoes, raspberries, strawberries, red peppers, and red onions, for example, get their hues from lycopene, a powerful antioxidant that mops up cell-damaging free radicals and cuts the risk of certain cancers, including breast and cervical cancers. Orange foods like carrots, sweet potatoes, and mangos are filled with alpha- and beta-carotene, which the liver converts to vitamin A and retinol, key nutrients needed for eye health, immune defenses, and healthy cell division. Green foods—think kale, spinach, and broccoli—are loaded with nutrients that detoxify the body and help you lose weight. Blue and purple foods such as blueberries, blackberries, and beets contain health-protective antioxidants.

When you eat a plateful of colorful foods, the nutrients act synergistically to combat disease. The phytochemicals in the red strawberries you ate for breakfast, for instance, may fight off illness more effectively when combined with the mashed avocado on your morning toast. If you can prep your meals with at least three colors each, you're on your way to the healthiest, leanest, and most vibrant body ever.

I don't want you thinking that I am trying to convert you into a vegan, though! The proof is in the science that eating plant-based is healthier for the planet, your body, and your waistline. My goal throughout this book is to provide incredibly delicious, real food recipes. These recipes are predominantly plant-based, but my goal is to get you to include more fruits, vegetables, and plant-based proteins. There is no converting here and no judgment either way.

My 28-Day Meal Prep Weight-Loss Plan

All of this brings me to my 28-day plan that you'll be following here. Here's how you'll do it:

- You'll eat three main meals—breakfast, lunch, and dinner—in moderate but filling serving sizes.
- You'll enjoy two optional snacks daily. You have the option of prepping some scrumptious snacks for the week, or keep it simple with fresh fruit and nuts.
- You have the option of eating one luscious but nutritious dessert each week; choose one day and make a plan to whip up the dessert you choose from the recipes provided.
- You'll have plenty of vegetables, fruits, nuts, grains, and seeds. But you don't have to stick with 100 percent plants. For those who want to take a stepwise approach to the plan, you can add in animal protein foods such as eggs, poultry, fish, or meat. There are a few recipes throughout the book that do include some of these items, and you can either follow those, swap out the animal products with vegan ones, or skip the recipe altogether and pick a different one you like.
- You'll eat one mainly raw meal daily, such as one of my colorful

salads with loads of extras on top that will leave you nourished and satisfied.

- You'll be introduced to "souping," a healthier alternative to juicing.
- You won't eat dairy and you will consume minimal salt, but you'll find that you won't miss either, because you'll be using *delicious* nut milks and you'll discover how to season your foods so that they taste better spiced than salted.
- You'll get your share of healthy, beneficial fats from nuts, seeds, and good-for-you oils such as coconut oil and olive oil.
- You'll drink plenty of liquids—water (including my detox waters), smoothies, and herbal teas.

So that's an overview of the plan. It's divided into four weeks, and each week has a different theme, so you never get bored. Changing this up is also good for your body—by varying your meals and their flavor, you continue giving your body everything it needs for healthy weight loss.

Week One: Cleansing Soups and Healing Smoothies

Unlike juice cleanses, which are loaded with natural sugar from fruit and contain no fiber, soups contain little sugar, so you avoid blood sugar spikes that can leave you feeling moody, tired, and craving sugar. Vegetable "souping" lets you have a calorie-light day full of healthy ingredients *while still getting fiber*. A steaming bowl of soup not only warms you up but is a fast and efficient way to pack nutrients into your diet.

I've found soup to be a delicious weight-loss tool too. Soup is largely liquid and can satisfy your appetite. With water-rich foods like soup, you'll feel full and be less likely to get overly hungry, slip up, or binge. In a 2005 study conducted at Pennsylvania State University for *Obesity Research,* researchers reported that overweight or obese women who consumed two daily servings of soup lost 50 percent more weight than dieters who did not eat soup but had two snacks instead.

You'll also be adding smoothies into week one, using my favorite smoothie recipes. They taste amazing, and they're high in fiber and healthy fats. Like soups, smoothies are a wonderful weight-loss tool because they keep you feeling full despite the fact that you're consuming fewer calories.

Plus, a week of soups and smoothies gives your digestive system a break, because the nutrients are absorbed and assimilated into your body much more easily than they would be from solid food. This means fewer hunger pangs, more energy, and natural weight loss without ever looking at a label or counting calories.

That's week one: the souping and smoothie phase. After these first seven days, expect to be pleasantly surprised when you step on the scale. Based on what I've observed with my clients, you'll probably be lighter by about 5 pounds or more.

Week Two: Fiber Up

In week two, you'll up the fiber ante. I find fiber to be one of the best weight-loss weapons in the world because of its influence on insulin control, hunger, and body fat storage. Beans, chickpeas, peas, and lentils are among the foods highest in fiber—and they pack a punch for weight loss and weight control, as reported by Canadian researchers in 2016 in the *American Journal of Clinical Nutrition*. They analyzed data from twenty-one clinical trials on these fiber-packed foods and found that they can help dieters shed unwanted pounds and reduce body fat—all without counting calories or restricting other foods. The analysis also showed that people eating these foods did not gain weight back after losing it.

The Canadian team also reported that these foods have a low glycemic index—meaning that they break down gradually in the digestive tract and the fiber may reduce the absorption of fat too. They also appear to help lower blood levels of LDL ("bad") cholesterol.

There's more good news: eating beans, chickpeas, peas, and lentils makes people feel fuller. Of course, this is key to weight loss. One reason I believe that so many diets fail is because people suffer from hunger and food cravings, which makes a diet unsustainable.

Conversely, trouble starts when we eat low-fiber foods: refined carbs, like those found in white bread, cake, cookies, and other baked goods. These foods are practically devoid of fiber and thus quickly digested, activating a rapid spike in blood glucose. In reaction, the pancreas churns out lots of insulin to wipe up the surplus glucose, though some of it will likely get packed away as fat. Then blood glucose levels fall to the point where you feel so shaky, you're crazy to eat again.

The foods I emphasize on this plan are fiber-rich, non-processed, and lower-glycemic carbohydrates. They don't elicit the same kind of spike-and-crash response, and they make you feel full, so you don't overeat. In addition to beans, you'll also up your consumption of veggies like broccoli, leafy greens, cauliflower, cucumbers, and celery—along with nutritious grains, nuts, and seeds.

An important note: You won't be choosing boxed foods with labels that say "high fiber." Those products are usually made with wood pulp (typically labeled as "cellulose") after the real fiber has been naturally removed. You're going to eat foods naturally high in fiber—not splinters or anything termites eat!

So that's week two, the fiber-up phase.

After both weeks, expect to be around 5 to 10 pounds lighter than you are right now. Seriously! This weight will drop from every part of your body . . . so start anticipating a flatter tummy and thinner thighs. But these aren't the only changes you'll experience. Your body will love the surge of nutrients it's receiving—so you'll find that you're more energetic, in a better mood, sleeping well throughout the night, and experiencing an overall feeling of well-being. And believe me, the time you spend prepping your meals on Sunday will free up the rest of the week to unleash your newfound energy on activities you enjoy or felt too tired to cross off your to-do list!

Week Three: The Protein Period

Protein is to your body what a wood frame is to your house or steel is to a bridge. Nutritionally, it's the most important structural material in your body, vital to exceptional health because of its role in building, repairing, and maintaining the body.

If you don't get enough protein, your body will start breaking down muscle tissue to yield energy and you'll lose body-firming muscle, which will sabotage your weight-loss efforts.

I'm well aware that low-carb, high-protein diets are all the rage, and they can be an effective way to lose weight. But on my plan, you will increase your protein intake mostly from plants such as beans and legumes, which also happen to be higher in carbohydrates than animal proteins. Will you still lose weight? Yes! In 2014, researchers from the School of Public Health at Loma Linda University in California compared weight loss in dieters who followed either a low-carb diet or a high-fiber legume diet. They found that the bean-rich diet worked as well as a low-carbohydrate diet for losing weight, with the added benefit of tamping down artery-clogging cholesterol, which often plagues low-carb, high-protein dieters. I like hearing that, because I'm all about having a healthy body first and foremost. Health is wealth, after all.

In terms of satisfying hunger, protein is more effective than the other macronutrients and requires more energy to break down and assimilate. And whereas carbs can spike your blood sugar and insulin, protein does not. Having plant-based proteins such as beans gives you a high protein-to-fiber-to-carbohydrate ratio, making it one of the healthiest foods on the planet. So don't worry about carbohydrates and a lack of protein on this plan. It is designed to keep you full, help you drop the weight, and improve your digestion.

The U.S. Centers for Disease Control recommend 50 grams of protein daily, which you'll easily get as long as you eat the beans, nuts and seeds, grains, and vegetables that I recommend. As I've pointed out, plant protein is as effective as animal protein for losing and managing weight, building and preserving muscle, and making the stuff our bodies need for good health. Just look at a horse (a plant-eater) and you'll be reassured that plant proteins build sleek, lean muscle, and plenty of it. Still not convinced? I challenge you to try out the protein power week with the recipes written as they are and see how you feel. I'm certain you will have more energy, will have better digestion, and will find yourself thinking more clearly. Remember, you still have the option to add animal products, so follow the plan as best you can and modify as needed.

So that's week three, the protein phase. More good news: the number on the scale is dropping. Don't be surprised if you're down by 8 to 15 pounds by the end of the third week. And I'm sure your clothes are fitting better too, not to mention that your tummy is going to be flatter.

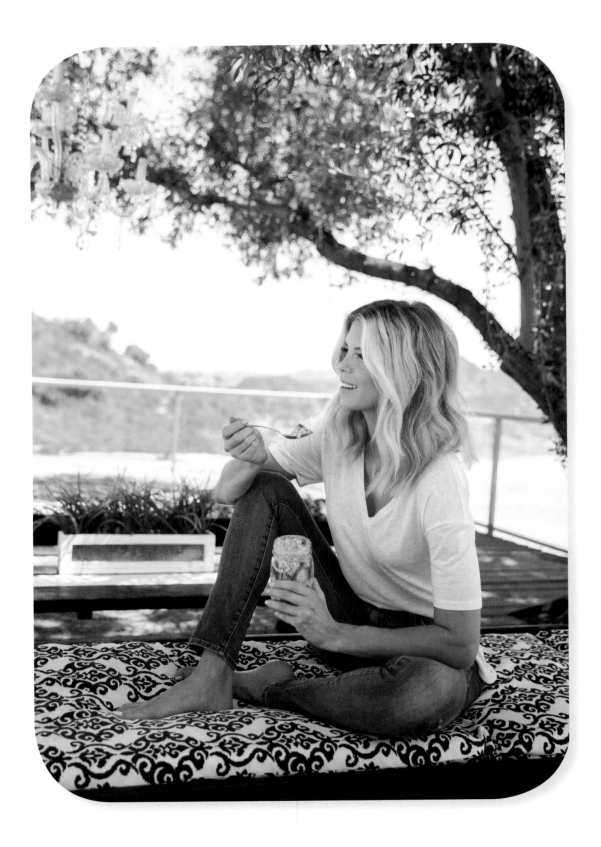

Week Four: Detox

Finally, in week four, you'll eat foods and enjoy recipes that emphasize known "detox foods." These foods naturally detox your body to help you lose additional weight, break through a plateau, and, for many of you, shed those last 5 stubborn pounds.

Detoxification is the process of cleansing toxins from the body. When I mention "toxins," I'm talking about the pesticides, artificial hormones, additives, and preservatives with which our food is treated, as well as the excess sugar, alcohol, caffeine, tobacco, pharmaceutical drugs, air pollution, bacteria, and viruses to which our bodies are routinely exposed—either by our lifestyle choices or through the environment.

According to the American Academy of Environmental Medicine, there are some ninety thousand chemicals commonly circulating in the modern world, many of which may produce chemical sensitivities, ranging from allergies to chronically poor health. When chemicals don't break down fast enough or the body's processes can't keep up with intake, you can develop a variety of symptoms; everything from weight gain, aches and pains, headaches, dull skin, acne, lack of energy, insomnia, constipation, and bloating to cellulite, joint pain, depression, and severe fatigue. As if these aren't enough reasons to detox, a buildup of toxins is also associated with diseases such as fibromyalgia, Parkinson's, Alzheimer's, and cancer, just to name a few.

I'm sure you've heard the back-and-forth on whether detoxing is actually good for you. One side says it's all nonsense: your body does a beautiful job of cleansing and detoxifying itself. But detox advocates say our bodies need to be flushed with the help of juice cleanses and water fasts, which reset our metabolism, our gut health, and nearly every other system in our body.

So, what's the truth here? Well, for more details on this I highly recommend you check out my first book, *The 5-Day Real Food Detox,* in which I talk all about detoxing. The short of it, though, is that yes, our bodies naturally detox, and our liver is an incredible organ of detoxification. However, we are exposed to so many chemicals in our food supply and in the environment that the body becomes overwhelmed and needs the nudge of an occasional detox. Simply put, a detox is good for your body and health, because you're essentially cutting out unhealthy foods and

17

drinks and replacing them with nutrient-rich ones. This is what detoxing really means to me. It's not about anything other than removing something not as good for you, say alcohol, and replacing it with something better for you—a green smoothie, for instance. There is not a single person who can argue that having a bit less booze and a bit more fruits and veggies isn't healthy. So think of the detoxing week as just adding in more beneficial things to your body.

What are those foods? Think beets, cruciferous veggies, avocados, fennel, raw spinach, onions, beans, garlic, and red peppers. While not technically a detox or a cleanse, this week will teach you about cleansing foods, and it's a great way to finish out the four weeks, breaking any plateau you might have and leaving you feeling lighter than you ever imagined.

That's week four, the detox phase.

After 28 days, a lot of changes have taken place. You've lost weight, steadily and naturally—perhaps up to 15 to 20 pounds total. Your body is responding positively to the alterations in your diet. You're experiencing less bloating and fewer cravings. Your skin is clear, and your energy levels are so high that you don't even miss your unhealthy indulgences.

So, you can have the body—and brain—you want by solidifying your meal prep habits and increasing plant foods in your diet. You just have to . . .

Secret #3: Be Consistent

What we do on a daily basis is more important than what we do once in a blue moon. Consistency is the key, my friends. Without it, your progress will stall.

How can you stay consistent? First, focus on making small healthy choices each day. It's these changes that add up to the big ones you ultimately desire. Second, don't beat yourself up if you slip. Just get back on the plan and keep moving forward. Third, put in the work. If you eat healthy only occasionally, you won't develop a rockin' bod.

I'd like you to remember one thing going forward, though. This book is all about consistency. The more you do the meal prep, the easier it will become. The first time you do it, you might find it frustrating or time consuming. But I promise that it will become easier, just like riding a bike or driving a car. The more we do something, the easier it becomes. So stick with it even if it's hard, and the rewards will become apparent.

The other thing I'd like you to take away from this is that everything is customizable to you! If you hate tomatoes, please do not feel compelled to eat them. I receive countless questions from people thinking that they cannot make a certain recipe of mine because it has one ingredient they don't like. What I'd like you to take away from this book is that cooking is fun, meal prepping is easy and effective, and you will find things that work for your lifestyle. If you are fully vegan, then either skip the recipes that mention an animal product or swap it out for plant-based protein that you love. A recipe has almonds, and you can't have them? Use a different nut. The other thing to note is that if you absolutely think that the meal prep is going to be too much for the week or you don't want to make all the variations of meals, then simplify it. I always say, even if you cannot do a plan 100 percent, trying to do it is still better than not doing it at all!

There are definitely weeks that I know are going to be busier than others, whether it's a lot of meetings each day, or certain dinners I cannot avoid. When I hit these points, I absolutely simplify my meal prep to make sure that I am still going to eat the food I have in my fridge and not fall off-track. The key to simplifying the meal prep each week is making note of any recipes you would like to eat multiple days and buying extra ingredients for those, instead of what is written. For example, if you want to make this plan really simple, choose two breakfast options and alternate between them throughout the week, depending what week you're on. Do the same for lunch and dinner. The plan is written to give you an abundance of delicious recipes so you don't get bored; however, I don't want you getting overwhelmed and quitting altogether. It's better to eat a few recipes I've provided each week than none at all!

Now, before we dive into the mechanics of meal prepping, let's talk about the amazing ways it can help curb emotional overeating.

CHAPTER 2

Stop Emotional Overeating Through Meal Prepping

So many people turn to food to heal emotional problems, and I'm sure it contributes to our skyrocketing obesity statistics. You see, when we eat to satisfy emotional cravings, not physical ones, we usually end up making very unhealthy choices. (I have yet to meet someone who turns to kale when they're feeling down.) The typical emotional eater tends to consume "comfort" or junk food in large quantities in response to feelings, rather than hunger. And there's usually a trigger.

You get an upsetting text from your significant other or your mom, or maybe that person who you thought was going to call didn't. Work was really stressful, and traffic made you want to scream. You get home, and emotions take over. Out comes the food, and down it goes: the ice cream eaten at the end of a long and stressful day. An entire bag of chips consumed mindlessly. The package of cookies wolfed down during a good cry. A bottle of wine emptied in an attempt to ease stress. A huge fast-food meal gulped down during a nervous rant. Does this remind you of anyone? Well, it reminds me of how I used to be.

I'm going to share a little something with you here that I've never publicly admitted before. I have done all of the above—and more. From ages 19 to 27, I was anorexic; I starved myself so much that my bones were visible under my skin. Later, I developed binge eating disorder, a condition characterized by excessive overeating. Food became my enemy for many years. I was afraid of what it would do to my body. I went from full control (too much, in fact) to a complete loss of it in regard to food.

I was naturally skinny growing up, but, as I got older, I started to feel the pressures of keeping my impossibly small size, so I began dieting. Of course, our bodies naturally change shape with age. My body at age 12 was most definitely not supposed to be my body at age 19. But the media would like us to think otherwise. From a young age, we are bombarded with images and messages that make us feel we should look like teenagers.

Still, I continued to restrict my food intake and lost weight. Being skinny made me feel good.

Well, I got too skinny. People told me I actually needed to gain weight. It started while I was modeling in South Korea and was told to gain weight rapidly for certain jobs. So I ate Snickers, chips, and any other food that I'd previously avoided. Eating those foods didn't make me feel good, so although I did go back to eating less, I ate "real food," like lettuce, hard-boiled eggs, and, while I was in Seoul, steamed cabbage. Food was still the bad guy—but one that was ironically giving me comfort.

I won't go into how I overcame the two eating disorders—that's a whole book in itself—but I will say that through these experiences, I learned a lot about food and the way it can become linked to emotional hunger.

Cut to my gradual recovery from eating disorders: I still placed a lot of importance on food, the numbers on the scale, and stress. When I felt good, I would eat healthy and exercise. Life was dandy. But if I had one moment in that day when I felt bloated or fat, or I got upset from a

21

meeting, or I was too tired to exercise, I would end up bingeing. This vicious cycle went on and on, day after day.

While on a binge, I tumbled into a place of nothingness. I felt neither pain nor happiness. I was simply numbing myself with food. I felt good while I was eating, in a state of peace really, but only for about ten minutes. My "food euphoria" quickly wore off and was replaced with guilt over what I had eaten and how easily I had been triggered to eat it.

The following day, I'd restrict myself to eating almost nothing, or low-calorie veggies like lettuce all day long and nothing else, to make up for the binge. By evening though, I'd have the same crappy feelings about myself: I'd never be fit or look good, and so I'd binge again. The cycle kept going, and there was always an underlying emotion that made me binge: sadness, loneliness, anger, hurt, feeling unvalued, feeling *unworthy*.

See a pattern? Have you ever felt this way?

Don't worry. There are solutions.

Food, Stress, and Meal Prep

As you follow my plan, you'll discover that meal prep removes the emotional stress from eating and the negative thoughts that surround food. When you prep, you've already got healthy food ready to go—no fuss, no worrying about what goes into your body, and no long hours spent cooking during the week. You have removed "food stress" from your life.

You see, food stress—obsessing over what you eat and feeling guilty about it—is more detrimental to your body, weight, and health than any plate of lasagna, slice of cheesecake, or huge buttered dinner roll you eat. Here's why: The stress adversely affects your digestion, so your body can't digest food properly. The calories are more easily stored, rather than burned up. Plus, stress creates excess stomach acid, which many experts believe makes you crave even more food.

Stress also interrupts your sleep, causing insomnia or poor-quality sleep. This situation triggers the release of too much cortisol, the stress hormone that causes insulin resistance (in which your cells block the entry of glucose and insulin) and weight gain. What's more, poor sleep may affect other hormones such as ghrelin and leptin, which control appetite and hunger.

Stressing over food and other issues can cause depression, which is associated with elevated cortisol levels and weight gain. Depression can cause bingeing behaviors, especially in those with eating disorders, and a lot of people who are depressed are also less physically active. Studies show that when we're anxious, many of us indulge in foods that are higher in fat and sugar, which are usually extremely caloric.

So stop the food guilt and change your attitude toward what you eat. Let's say you go to a birthday party. Decide that you will enjoy some cake, and don't obsess over eating it. Have a small slice. Savor each bite. Enjoy the tastes and different textures. Take foods like cake off the forbidden list and put them on the occasional list. Doing so will eliminate food stress and the weight gain that accompanies it.

Break Through Emotional Overeating

Let's take a quick step back here for a second. Many people have become so obsessed and guilt-ridden over food that they suffer from severely disordered eating, whether it's anorexia, bulimia, or binge-eating disorder. I'm not a doctor, nor have I studied psychology or addictive behaviors, but I do know that if you want to recover from a full-blown eating disorder, it is possible. Here are some tips that helped me, and I truly believe they will help you too. Please consult your doctor if things are very serious, because I am not here to diagnose or treat you. I know what it's like to suffer from these disorders, and if you need professional help, please seek it out. These tips are also great for people who do not have an eating disorder, but would just like some extra support to be less fearful or confused about the food they eat.

Tip 1: Meal Prep Helps Prevent Binge Eating

Once I started meal prepping, I realized it helped to prevent and control emotional overeating and bingeing. It's hard to overeat or binge when you have delicious foods in your fridge prepped and ready to eat.

Let's say you're heading to the movies, and you know from experience that you'll be tempted by the large-sized popcorn with butter (and all those refills). Avoid temptation by prepping your own smaller portions of air-popped popcorn with coconut oil and nutritional yeast flakes at home and bring it in your bag, along with some bottled water with lemon slices inside.

Meal prep also helped me to structure my eating, since I always had breakfast, lunch, dinner, and snacks planned out and prepared. Structured eating has been used in countless treatment plans to help people overcome disordered eating.

THE SKINNY ON DISORDERED EATING

You might not think that you have an eating problem, which is probably true, but many people have a complicated or unhappy relationship to food and eating. If you've ever yo-yo dieted, counted calories, or wondered why you aren't losing weight even though you watch what you eat, then the tips in this chapter will help you. It's about getting real with yourself and saying, "You know what? I do not want to be scared of food anymore!"

So, why does structured eating work? Eating three meals and at least two snacks daily helps you move from chaotic eating to organized eating. This means eating at set times, with your pre-prepared meals. Most people who eat emotionally or have eating disorders do not believe they can eat three normal meals and maintain a normal weight, but they can. With structured meals, you can combat many detrimental habits, including starving, bingeing, and purging. Progressing from chaotic eating to organized eating is the first step to getting your body and mind back in balance—and the best way to structure eating is to prep meals.

If you aren't suffering from an eating problem but want to control your weight in a healthy way, meal prepping will help you do so. For one, you won't skip meals—something we might do because we often feel we don't have time to eat. But meal skipping, especially breakfast, has been linked to weight gain, poor appetite control, lack of nutrients, and a higher risk of diabetes and possibly other chronic diseases, according to a 2010 study published in *Critical Reviews in Food Science and Nutrition*. A Harvard study found those who regularly skipped breakfast had a 27 percent higher risk of a heart attack than those who ate a morning meal. If you meal prep, you're less likely to miss a good, healthy meal.

Meal skipping, emotional overeating, and disordered eating behaviors deprive our bodies of the healthy food and nutrients we need. We have to train ourselves to learn how to eat "normally" again (and for some, for the first time)—and meal prepping is key.

Tip 2: A Prep Trick to Naturally Control Cravings for Sweets

Many people have the urge to drown their sorrows in sugary sweets. When you are in full binge mode, you want pure white cane sugar . . . cookies, chocolate, you name it! But you can have your sweets and eat them too. Meet your new best friends: 70 percent dark chocolate, coconut water, and dried mango. I keep little packets of chocolate and mango around, along with bottles of coconut water—just to be prepared in case I hit a turbulent patch and find myself craving sugar.

When I was first recovering from my eating disorder, these foods were my saving grace. I didn't feel as guilty eating them. When the urge to binge struck, as it inevitably would, I'd head to the store and buy these three treats. They allowed me to eat sugary but healthier foods, they calmed my nervous system down, and they eased my desire to binge. One reason for this, at least for me, is that dried mango takes a while to chew, and since chewing helps dissipate anger and stress, this particular food is a great thing to eat if you're angry or stressed! The coconut water left me feeling full and refreshed, while also cleansing my palate, so I didn't desire anything else. As for the delectable dark chocolate? It's hard to eat a whole bar, so I would just eat it until I couldn't fathom having any more. I'll be honest: there were times that I would eat the entire bar of dark chocolate, but trust me when I say that after a full bar you don't really want any more chocolate! It's a far cry from milk chocolate, which is incredibly easy to overeat because of all the sugar.

Feel a binge coming on? Dark chocolate, coconut water, and mango. Make them your go-to items.

Tip 3: Change the Way You Look at Exercise

When I was in the worst of my binge-and-starve cycles, I'd stuff myself with massive amounts of food. The next day I wouldn't eat at all, but I'd go to the gym and pound my body for an hour or two.

I hated this behavior, so I decided to change my attitude. I made it a rule that I went to the gym only if I had eaten healthfully that day. I had to reframe my mindset: exercise was no longer a punishment. When I followed this rule, my bingeing decreased considerably.

Why did it work so well? You see, I was automatically removing a negative reinforcement and replacing it with a positive one. If I ate well and felt great, even a walk in the park made me feel that much better.

Change the way you look at exercise. It is not a burden or a hardship, as many people think. It offers you a world of mind and body benefits.

I challenge you to figure out why you don't like exercising. Is it because it makes you feel out of shape? Or are you embarrassed that you can't do the exercises properly? Or are you simply scared? If so, then you need to change your mindset. You've made exercise a negative and unpleasant activity in your life. Think about the positive aspects of working out: it makes you feel great, it helps you fit into your clothes, and your skin looks radiant. After a day of healthy eating and exercise, focus on one of these positives. Do this for a week or two, then watch your attitude about exercise change, and observe how seldom you overeat. Remember, to see positive results, we have to have positive behaviors.

Tip 4: Journal to Identify Your Emotional Triggers

While going through my eating disorder and battling pretty intense insomnia, I began to journal to clear my mind. As I look back, I realize journaling helped tremendously. Once you start writing down where you are, what you are eating, how you feel, and what brings you joy, you begin to find out very quickly what is triggering your emotional overeating. This is also highly recommended if you are finding yourself overly stressed, getting angry quickly, or unable to sleep. Keeping a daily gratitude journal is also highly recommended to help with weight loss, reducing stress, and becoming happier. Each day write five things you were grateful for, no matter how big or small.

Once I started journaling, I began to realize that I never felt worthy—for two reasons. The first was that I never thought my body was good enough when I was modeling. So I didn't eat—but then I didn't get jobs. My self-worth was tied to how I looked and what I weighed. My value depended on a number on a scale, rather than on who I was as a person.

Second, I discovered that loneliness made me binge. I didn't always have roommates, but when I did, we didn't necessarily get along. All the people I'd grown up with were in another country, and I didn't feel that I was bringing value to the world. I felt isolated and lonely.

It took me a lot of time and inner work to understand that loneliness comes from within ourselves, as do sadness and happiness. No one else can fix that. So try to figure out what triggers your desire to overeat. Once you identify your triggers, you can begin to target those moments and fill them with positive actions. I used to binge on a Sunday night when I sat home all weekend, but my Sunday evenings changed when I started going to a yoga class where I knew people, or going to the movies, or inviting people over—and, of course, meal prepping.

Tip 5: Don't Just Allow a Binge to Happen; Make It a Beautiful Binge

I know what you're thinking—I'm crazy to suggest this. But stay with me. You and I both know that trying to control yourself when you're about to go into full-on binge mode doesn't work. If you've never binged and haven't

27

experienced this, then you're lucky. But if you know you're going to binge, don't stop it. Decide exactly what you want to have and have it. Let's take pizza, for example, because one of the last times I binged, it was on pizza. Instead of getting a crappy pizza from a fast-food chain, I went to a specialty pizza shop and ordered three ginormous slices. They packed them up for me, and I bought a bottle of very nice red wine. When I got home, I reheated the slices, poured myself a glass of wine, set a nice tray out on my table in front of my couch, lit some candles, and turned on my favorite TV show. I sat calmly eating that pizza and sipping the wine while enjoying my show.

Basically, I created a mindful, meaningful binge, rather than one in which I was wolfing down crappy food until I felt numb, guilty, and depressed. Okay, I didn't exactly feel amazing the next day, because all that pizza I ate definitely took a toll on my body, but I had savored the food in a loving way. I'm not saying that you won't have some bad feelings the next day, but they'll start to become less intense.

Remember, you are in control; food is not. You'll begin to realize you feel good when you reward yourself with exercise instead of punishing yourself. And you can overcome a binge by simply allowing it to be a romantic dinner for one (or two, if your dog is there), with candles, your favorite movie, and your binge food, which is no longer called that—*just call it dinner.*

One More Important Point . . .

What should you do if you find yourself cheating during the 28 days?

I'd like you to go back and read this whole section again, especially Tip 4. Identify your triggers. Is there something going on in your life that is causing you discomfort or emotional pain? It might be anything from "I feel fat" to "I'm scared I will lose my job," plus a whole range of other emotions and negative self-talk.

So journal every time you start to feel a binge coming on and write down what triggered it. Did your boss yell at you? Did your man not text back? Do you feel bloated? When you write enough of these down, you'll begin to see a pattern.

If you binge-eat after looking in the mirror because you're unhappy with how you look, you are basing your self-worth on external things. What would I do in this situation? Write myself positive sticky notes and place them all over my mirror each time I say I don't like myself for one reason or another. Write yourself notes about your gorgeous brown hair, your beautiful strong arms, your lovely manicured fingernails, and so forth. Again, you're replacing negatives with positives, and your self-respect will grow. I love to put bright sticky notes all over my mirror to remind myself of the qualities I like.

The point of all this is not to say that bingeing or cheating is okay or not okay. Nor am I trying to give you an excuse to go off the plan. I'm giving you the tools that I wish I'd had when I was suffering through two eating disorders and trying to overcome hard-core body dysmorphia (an obsessive, flawed preoccupation with appearance).

I'm sharing these tools with you because I know they work. I was the guinea pig, and now I teach my methods to my clients. Today, these clients binge far less often than they used to, and many have completely stopped, and they know that meal prepping is an important step toward restoring organized eating. And remember, if you do end up cheating or bingeing, just continue the plan as normal. Don't try to modify the meals and skip carbs; simply stick to the plan.

Today is a new day. A new beginning. You have the power to change anything that isn't working for you. Meal prep will help you make the changes you need to break the cycle and start your beautifully healthy and happy life.

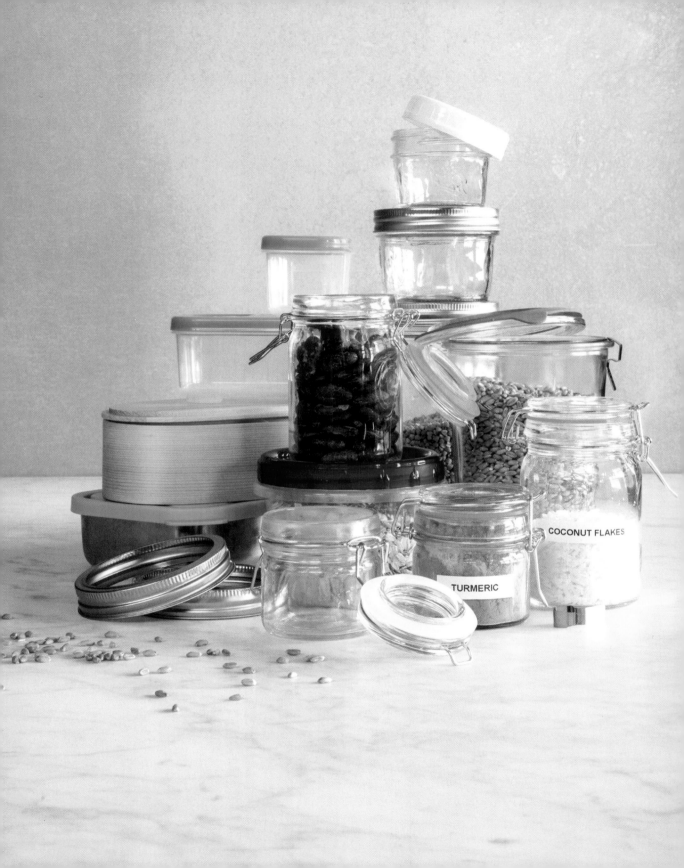

CHAPTER 3

The Power of Prep

Do you feel like you're too busy to spend time in the kitchen preparing healthy food that will help you lose weight? Are your portion sizes sometimes out of control?

I've got encouraging news for you: You do have time to cook, and you don't have to spend hours every day doing it. And you can eat nutritiously, control your portions, and get healthy and fit. You just need to use my system of meal prepping, in which preparing and cooking happen seamlessly.

Meal prepping might seem daunting initially, but I assure you, it makes eating healthy and losing weight an effortless decision. I'm going to show you how, week by week. But first, here are some simple overall strategies to make this time-saving trick work for you.

Plan: Get Your Kitchen Prep Ready

First things first! Planning is essential when it comes to meal prep. It ensures that you don't just go to the store and pick up random ingredients you'll never use.

Containers

Part of planning involves having a variety of containers on hand for your meal prep. Make sure you have quality leakproof and airtight containers so you don't end up with messes and spills. Buy containers of all sizes too. Small containers are perfect for snacks and salad dressings. If you're making salad dressings, save yourself some serious time and aggravation by preparing one batch and dividing it into these small containers. That way you can drizzle some dressing over your salad, or fork-dip when you're ready to eat. Snack-sized plastic baggies also help you measure out the perfect, ready-to-eat portions of seeds, nuts, vegetable sticks, and other snacks.

Find containers that are easy to stack in your fridge and are microwave, freezer, and dishwasher safe too. You'll save space in your fridge and time on cleanup.

I love using mason jars for salads and smoothies, and for storing super grains and super ingredients. They are great, because they are clear, so it's easy to see what's in them, and because they're microwave friendly. As for plastic containers, make sure they are BPA free. BPA is used to harden plastics, and it can be toxic to the body. Leached BPA has been linked to a host of health problems, including cancer, reproductive dysfunction, and heart disease.

Bento boxes and stainless steel lunch boxes work very well for packed lunches. Bento boxes are containers with separate compartments for proteins, grains, vegetables, and other components of your meal. For meal preppers, they are the best lunch boxes.

Kitchen Tools

Here's a look at what you might need in your kitchen for meal prepping. This list might seem intimidating at first, but when you look closely you'll realize that you already have most of these things.

Which are the most important items and which are optional? Although a spiralizer is not mandatory, I personally love it and highly recommend you get one. On the other hand, you can skip getting both a food processor and a blender, and instead go for a high-speed blender that has both capabilities. My favorite ones? High-end products are Blendtec and Vitamix; low end, the Ninja. There's no need to go buy top-of-the-line equipment at first. Start with something cheaper. If you use it a lot, then upgrade later.

If you have room in your kitchen, the slow cooker is an exceptional piece of equipment. You can add beans and water, set the timer, and come back when they're done. It makes cleanup much easier, and you save money by purchasing dried goods instead of canned.

All the recommended items here are exactly that: recommended and not mandatory. You won't necessarily use every single item in the coming recipes, so pick and choose which ones are most useful to you when starting the plan. Here are other kitchen tools to consider:

Utensils

Mixing spoons

Wooden spoons

Spatula

Chef's knife

Can opener

Cutting board

Grater

Measuring spoons and cups

Mixing bowl

Cookware

Skillets (large and small)

Saucepans (large and small)

Baking trays

Parchment paper

Baking dishes

Silicone or tin loaf pan; 8 ½ x 4 ½ inches

Slow cooker

Containers/Storage

Mason jars, 16-ounce

Mason jars, 16-ounce wide
 mouth

Airtight glass canisters

Zip-top baggies

Glass meal prep containers

Plastic containers, BPA-free

Bento lunch box or stainless
 steel lunch box

Extras

Masking tape and marker (for
 labeling)

Silicone food covers

Food processor

High-speed blender

Vegetable peeler

Melon baller

Spiralizer

Steamer basket

Mandoline slicer

Write It Out

Grab a notebook and pen or access a blank note page on your iPad. It's time to start mapping out your meals for the week. My 28-day meal plan will help you, but here are a few general pointers.

Look at your week and see which days require you to have all your meals fully prepped and ready to go. Check your calendar for special events. If you know you have a business lunch on Wednesday that will provide food, skip prepping that meal so that no food goes to waste. Then think about who in your family needs which meals, and how many servings you'll need. If you're single, or cooking for just two, meal prep is super easy.

Also, figure out which day is the best to prep. You can prep on Sunday for Monday through Wednesday, then prep again on Wednesday for the rest of the week. I have found that dividing it into these two days saves the most time and is effective for having meals on hand. If you follow me on social media, you know that Sunday afternoon I always make hummus, cook my beans, boil lentils, cook quinoa, and get my snacks ready for the week. I love to put on music and make prepping an enjoyable experience.

Shop

On my plan, you'll be eating certain recipes each day and each week. Take a moment to look over those recipes at the start of the week. I've provided weekly shopping lists that are organized into staples such as spices, vegetables, fruits, grains, and additional foods.

Because Sunday is a logical prep day for many people, it's also a good day to purchase any foods you need for the upcoming week. A few things to keep in mind:

- Check your pantry and fridge for items that you already have.
- Note any recipes that you may want to double or triple, or ones that you are omitting that week.
- Make sure to include all ingredients in your list (unless you already have them on hand).
- Take your shopping list to the supermarket or farmer's market, check each item off, and stick to the list. I suggest that you shop after a meal to ensure you're not hungry and tempted by extra purchases.

BUDGET SAVER
TIP #1: BUY IN BULK

When meal prepping, it's a good idea to buy some foods in bulk. Bulk purchases are less expensive and are free of salt, sugar, and chemicals used to keep the packaged products fresh. Stores such as Safeway and Kroger allow shoppers to bring their own tubs and fill them with dried goods: nuts, beans, cereals, and rice, for example. I always recommend grabbing around ½ pound of any type of dried goods. See how rapidly you use it up. If it goes fast, then you need to buy bigger quantities the next time out. This saves a lot of money and reduces trash.

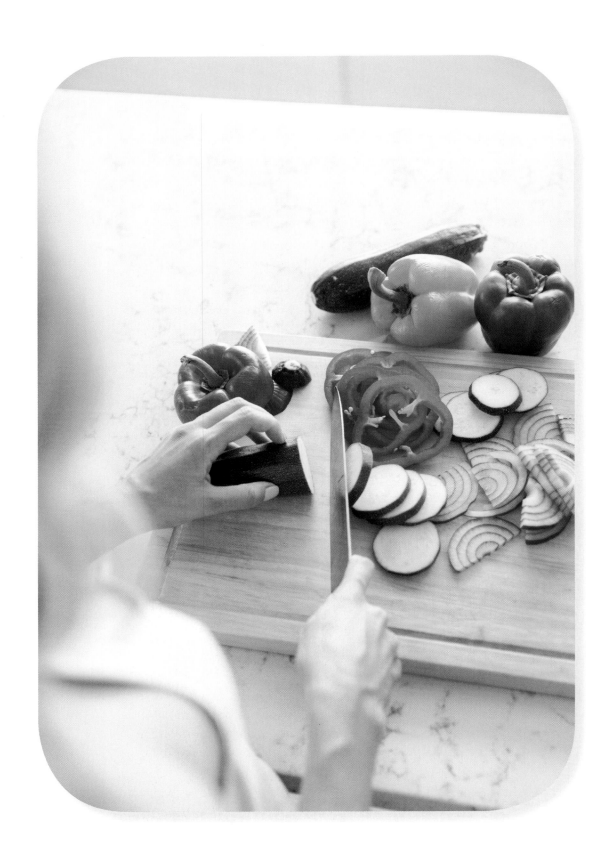

Basic Prep: Some Assembly Required

Now it's time to prep! You'll be able to fully prepare most of these recipes right away and pack them in the fridge or freezer. For your prep:

- Clear enough worktop space, particularly near the oven and microwave. Kitchen islands are great meal prep areas.
- Gather together your gadgets, utensils, and containers. Have a heavy, wide chef's knife on hand to cut tough vegetables.
- Have an order for your prep operation. For example, start with foods that require the longest to cook, like rice and potatoes. This will take some trial and error.
- Wash your hands thoroughly prior to prepping any food.

Fruit, Veggie, Grains, and Smoothie Prep

- Wash and chop all raw vegetables and place them in bags for salads. Alternatively, you can purchase washed and bagged lettuce, or pre-chopped onions, bell peppers, or other veggies. These usually come in their own containers or bags.
- Spiralizing lets you prep vegetables in seconds, and turn them into no-carb "noodles." There are several types of spiralizers on the market; all work well and are inexpensive. When you spiralize vegetables, such as zucchini, you're increasing your healthy options for that week. Instead of a side of sliced zucchini, for example, you can prepare a large bowl of Zucchini Noodles with Hemp Pesto. Delicious!
- Roast different vegetables together that have the same cooking time. Roasting vegetables brings out their natural sweetness, but it takes 30 to 40 minutes for each pan of nutrient-rich goodness to roast. To prep a large batch of veggies, pair them based on compatible roasting times. Faster-cooking vegetables that can be

baked in the same pan include asparagus, mushrooms, and cherry tomatoes; slower-cooking vegetables include carrots, Brussels sprouts, cauliflower, and potatoes.

- Learn to blanch veggies. Blanching is an easy and affordable way to prep and store a large portion of vegetables while maintaining their nutritional value. To blanch, simply steam or boil veggies for approximately 2 to 3 minutes until their color becomes slightly brighter, then quickly transfer them to a bowl of cold water with ice (this stops the cooking process so that the veggies remain firm and vibrant when you reheat them). Remove the veggies after they have cooled down, shake off any excess water, and place them on a rack with a towel underneath to release a bit more water before putting them in containers.

  Blanched vegetables can be portioned and frozen for months. No need to buy store-bought frozen vegetables (unless you want to)—you can now make your own.

- Steam veggies. This is one of the easiest and healthiest ways to prep vegetables. Cut veggies into bite-sized pieces. Insert a steamer basket into the pot and add about an inch of water under the basket. Bring the water to a boil over high heat. Add veggies to the basket, cover, and reduce heat to medium. Your veggies are done when they are vibrantly colored and tender.

  You can steam veggies in your microwave too. Place them in a microwave-safe dish. Add a little water to the bottom, cover with plastic wrap, and leave one corner open to vent.

- Cook certain grains ahead of time so you can quickly warm them up or use them cold in salads. Rice actually freezes well. Cook a large quantity, portion it, and freeze. You won't have to cook rice for a couple of weeks if you do this.

- Pre-portion smoothie ingredients in a plastic, freezable baggie and pop them in your freezer. All that's left for you to do in the morning is to blend the contents with water, coconut water, or nut milk and pour the healthy goodness into a to-go cup if you need to hit the road.

  Another one of my tricks is to make smoothie "ice cubes." Blend

DIFFERENT VEGETABLES HAVE DIFFERENT STEAM TIMES ON THE STOVE

2 to 5 minutes	5 to 7 minutes	7 to 10 minutes	10 to 15 minutes
Spinach	Asparagus	Brussels sprouts	Onions
Peas	Broccoli	Carrots	Potatoes, grated
	Cauliflower	Green beans	
	Kale	Squash	

together veggies and fruit; pour the mixture into an ice cube tray and freeze. Add these to your smoothies later on, rather than use ice. Both techniques make drinking healthy smoothies hassle-free and save you plenty of time.

- Enjoy my Overnight Oats (page 219). These are great to make in the evening, so you can grab and go in the morning when you don't have a lot of time.

QUICK GUIDE TO ROASTING VEGETABLES

1. Preheat oven to 425°F.
2. Chop pieces into similar sizes, such as 1-inch squares for butternut squash and potatoes, Brussels sprouts in half, etc.
3. Toss chopped vegetables with 1 tablespoon of olive oil and add a pinch of salt and pepper if desired. Mix with hands to cover all pieces.
4. Spread evenly over a parchment lined baking tray without overcrowding the tray.

10 to 15 minutes	15 to 20 minutes	20 to 25 minutes	25 to 30 minutes	35 to 40 minutes
Mushrooms	Squash	Tomatoes	Onions	Broccoli
	Asparagus	Bell peppers	Eggplant	Sweet potatoes
	Brussels sprouts		Carrots	Butternut squash
			Cauliflower	White potatoes
				Beets

If you're a keen budgeter yet have a taste for all things organic, then fruit and veggie boxes could be for you. However, if you don't mind non-organic produce, purchasing fruits and veggies at your supermarket will be the far cheaper option. Here's the deal, however: an organic food box from a supplier, delivered to your doorstep, can be about 20 percent cheaper than supermarket organic brands. For the best buys, check out these companies: Gousto, Farm Fresh to You, and Mama Earth. Companies such as Imperfect Produce in California are also wonderful options—and are economical.

Protein Prep

- Hard-boil eggs. These are an excellent source of protein, vitamins, and good fats, and therefore make terrific on-the-go snacks. There are two foolproof ways to hard-boil eggs.

  On the stove: Fill a large saucepan with cold water. Place the eggs in the water, along with 1 teaspoon vinegar, and put the pan on your stove. Turn the burner on high and bring to a boil. Turn the heat off, cover, and allow the eggs to rest in the hot water for 15 minutes. If your stove doesn't retain heat well, keep the burner on low. Afterward, drain the pan and refill it with ice water. Let the eggs sit for 5 minutes; drain and refrigerate.

  In the oven: Hard-boil eggs in the oven—not in a pot. Place your eggs in muffin tins without water, and bake at 350 degrees for just 30 minutes.

  Ta-da! Both methods give you a perfectly hard-boiled batch.

- Pre-cook poultry and other meats if you are going to have animal protein as part of your meals. Prep extra chicken or other meat to have protein on hand to add into salads, sandwiches, or wraps. (Most of my recipes are plant-based, but they can be easily adjusted for the addition of lean poultry, beef, fish, or other animal proteins.) Make sure you keep an eye on your animal proteins once they are in the fridge as they do not last as long as plant-based proteins.

- Try stir-fries. If you're planning a stir-fry, chop all the veggies and store them in one container. Slice the chicken, fish, shellfish, or meat (if using) and store it in another container. On the night you want to stir-fry, all you have to do is take out the containers and dump everything into a skillet or wok.

- To cut cooking time, buy a rotisserie chicken from the supermarket deli. Remove all the skin and pull the meat off the bones. Use the chicken in various recipes.

- Try canned chicken or tuna for a time-saving source of pre-cooked protein. (Check for sodium content first, and choose low-sodium products.) While none of the recipes call for tuna in this plan, it can be a good source of protein to add once a week.

BUDGET SAVER
TIP #3: BUY CHEAPER CUTS OF MEAT

Maybe you're not 100 percent sold on the plant-based way of eating yet. That's okay; my goal is to empower you with knowledge to help you on your journey to living a healthier lifestyle. For my carnivore friends, here are some ways to save money on meat. I always recommend purchasing organic meats and other animal products. It is better to have a higher quality organic piece of meat (fish, chicken, and eggs) less often, then eating conventional every day.

- Choose cooking methods that get the most flavor from cheaper meats. These include stewing, making casseroles, and using slow cookers.
- Save on chicken. Buying a whole chicken can sometimes cost you the same as buying just two chicken breasts. So why not purchase

a whole chicken, roast it, and enjoy your chicken breast with a side of steamed veggies? Make a chicken stew with the leftovers the next night. Then use any other leftover meat in a stir-fry the third night. Don't toss that carcass either. Boil it gently for a few hours to yield a tasty broth that can serve as a soup base. Or you can freeze the broth for later use.

- Beef: Purchase cheaper cuts such as the shin, leg, shank, or flank. These can be stewed, roasted, slow-cooked, or baked.
- Fish: Mackerel is often thought of as a "fishy" fish. But paired with arugula, beets, tomatoes, onion, and balsamic dressing in a salad, it's divine (and cheap!). Other cheaper fish include sardines, smoked haddock, and tuna. Just be sure they're farmed in an environmentally friendly way and not exposed to toxic conditions, or choose wild-caught fish. A great resource for this information is www.seafoodwatch.org. This organization publishes an extensive chart on the best and worst seafood choices.
- Lamb: Cuts on the bone tend to be cheaper and hold the most flavor. Next time you're in the grocery store, pick up a bone-in piece of lamb, sear it, and cook it in a slow cooker with sweet potatoes, prunes, apricots, butternut squash, chopped tomatoes, chickpeas, and Moroccan spices for a delicious tajine. Serve it over quinoa rather than couscous, and enjoy a salad on the side.

Refrigeration Tips

- Keep prepped salads fresh. I portion ingredients into my meal prep containers for at least five days' worth of salads. In order to keep your salad crisp, add one paper towel (folded over) on top of the ingredients in your salad container. This does two things: it soaks up any excess moisture that makes lettuce soggy, and it preserves the lettuce's crunch longer. You can do something similar with celery—wrap it in aluminum foil to prevent it from getting limp and soggy.
- Keep fresh herbs fresh for the week. Wrap them in damp paper

towels and place them in a plastic bag. Store the bag in the produce bin in your refrigerator. They will stay fresh for three to four days.

- Refrigerate your cooked meals within two hours of cooking. The sooner you get them stored, the longer they stay fresh. Don't put hot containers into the fridge, however. Allow the food to cool to room temperature; otherwise, it can throw off the temperature in your fridge, which can cause other foods to spoil.

- Refrigerate uncooked meat on the bottom shelf of the refrigerator; this is the coldest part of the fridge.

- Store eggs and condiments in the door bins; this is where the refrigerator temperature fluctuates most due to opening and closing.

- Use your crisper bin for storing fruits and veggies.

- Try to not stuff your fridge—the air can't circulate properly or keep the food at a safe temperature.

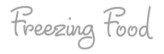

Freezing Food

When prepping for the week, make sure you follow safe freezing guidelines. For example:

- Keep your fridge temperature at 40°F or below and your freezer at 0°F or below. The temperatures of your refrigerator and freezer, as well as the types of containers you use, help preserve the freshness of your meals.

- Fully cook hot meals ahead of time; when the food is cool, place it in containers, allow to cool, and then refrigerate or freeze. Remember to do this in single-serve portions for portion control and less food waste.

- Make soups ahead of time. Soups can be frozen either in single servings or as a full batch.

- If you're going to freeze your meals, the containers must be airtight. If not, the food might get freezer burn and develop off flavors.

- Cool foods prior to freezing.
- Store oven-made meals in aluminum or glass containers with foil or plastic wrap on top.
- Store slow cooker meals in large plastic freezer bags. Remove as much air as possible and store them flat in your freezer.
- Place newer food packages in the back and move older frozen foods in front so they are next in line to be served.
- Freeze in smaller portions, if possible. This helps your food freeze and defrost faster—plus it allows for better portion control and less waste.
- Attach sticky notes or use masking tape with a Sharpie on your containers so that you can date each meal. This helps you reheat foods in the order they went into the freezer so they don't sit there for months.
- Freeze any leftovers. Then, by Wednesday or Thursday, when your energy and interest might be flagging, a pizza delivery doesn't necessarily spring to mind as the obvious dinner solution. There are already one or two components of a dish made and frozen, requiring only reheating.
- Know which foods freeze well and which ones don't:

Foods That Freeze Well

Meats, soups/stews, casseroles, slow cooker meals

Breads

Rice

Some fruits and vegetables (see table, page 46)

Herbs

Foods That Don't Freeze Well

Dairy (these foods will separate when frozen)

Foods with high water content (celery, lettuce, cucumbers)

Whole eggs

Cooked potatoes that aren't shredded

Pasta (unless slightly undercooked)

For more information and recipes for freezing, see Appendix A.

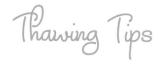

Thawing Tips

- I advise defrosting your meals in the fridge overnight for the next day. Be cautious if you're planning to use the microwave to defrost your meals. Sometimes the microwave heats up food too fast, and it can get overdone and dry; this can also deplete nutrients.
- Don't thaw foods at room temperature, to avoid the risk of spoilage and contamination.

Reheating Meals in the Microwave

- Use glass containers, or BPA-free plastic. Food can get so hot that it melts the plastic material, and substances and chemicals used in the manufacturing of the plastic can seep into your food and possibly be toxic if ingested.
- Cover your food with a damp paper towel to keep the food from drying out. Use this tip to keep your microwaved foods delicious.
- Don't microwave all your food at once. Chicken breasts, other animal proteins, and vegetables heat up at different speeds, so microwave heavier foods first and add lighter ones toward the end of the microwaving process.
- If you opt to not use your microwave for reheating, there are other options: convection ovens, ovens, stovetops, and rice cookers.

I've found that the best way to reheat food is to reheat it the same way it was cooked. Although it might not taste exactly the same, it'll be pretty close to it!

RECOMMENDED STORAGE TIMES FOR PROTEINS

Food	Refrigerator	Freezer
Eggs		
Eggs, fresh in shell	4–5 weeks	Don't freeze
Eggs, raw yolks/whites (separated)	2–4 days	1 year
Eggs, hard-boiled	1 week	Don't freeze
Egg substitutes, opened	3 days	Don't freeze
Egg substitutes, unopened	10 days	1 year
Meats and Poultry		
Frozen casseroles	—	3–4 months
Raw ground beef and stew meat	1–2 days	3–4 months
Raw ground turkey, veal, pork, lamb	1–2 days	3–4 months
Vegetable or meat-added soups/stews	3–4 days	2–3 months
Lean steaks	3–5 days	6–12 months
Cooked meat and meat dishes	3–4 days	2–3 months
Fresh chicken or turkey, whole	1–2 days	1 year
Fresh chicken, or turkey parts	1–2 days	9 months
Cooked poultry	3–4 days	4–6 months
Fish		
White fish	1–2 days	6 months
Fatty fish	1–2 days	2–3 months
Cooked fish	3–4 days	4–6 months
Fruits		
Apples	1 month	8–12 months
Apricots	3–5 days	8–12 months
Avocados	5 days	8–12 months
Bananas	5 days at room temperature	8–12 months
Berries	2–3 days	8–12 months
Cherries	2–3 days	8–12 months
Cranberries	1 week	8–12 months
Grapes	5 days	10–12 months
Guavas	1–2 days	8–12 months
Kiwis	6–8 days	4–6 months
Lemons, limes, oranges, grapefruits	2 weeks	4–6 months
Mangos	Ripen at room temperature	8–12 months
Melons	1 week	8–12 months
Nectarines	5 days	8–12 months
Papayas	Ripen at room temperature	8–12 months
Peaches	2–3 days	8–12 months
Pears	5 days	8–12 months

Pineapples	5–7 days	4–6 months
Plums	5 days	8–12 months
Vegetables		
Artichokes	2–3 days	Freeze poorly
Asparagus	2–3 days	8–12 months
Beets	2 weeks	8–12 months
Broccoli	3–5 days	8–12 months
Brussels sprouts	3–5 days	8–12 months
Cabbage	1 week	8–12 months
Carrots	2 weeks	8–12 months
Cauliflower	1 week	8–12 months
Celery	1 week	8–12 months
Corn (in husks)	1–2 days	8–12 months
Cucumbers	1 week	8–12 months
Eggplant	2–3 days	8–12 months
Green beans	1–2 weeks	8–12 months
Jicama	2–3 weeks	8–12 months
Lettuce and salad greens	3–5 days	Freeze poorly
Onions	1–2 weeks	4–6 months
Parsley	2–3 days	3–4 months
Peas	3–5 days	8–12 months
Peppers	1 week	8–12 months
Radishes	2 weeks	Freeze poorly
Squash, summer	3–5 days	8–12 months
Squash, winter	Store in a dry place	8–12 months
Tomatoes	1 week	8–12 months
Zucchini	3–5 days	8–12 months
Frozen vegetables	Do not refrigerate	8 months
Canned vegetables	1–4 days (opened)	2–3 months
Miscellaneous		
Bottled salad dressing	3 months	Freezes poorly
Coconut, shredded, open	8 months	1 year
Non-dairy milks	1 week	Freeze poorly
Nuts	6 months	1 year
Nut butter	6–8 months	6–8 months
Tofu	1 week	1 month
Yogurt	1 week after sell-by date	1–2 months

Sources: FDA.gov and the University of Kentucky, College of Agriculture

Additional Prep Tips

- Prep your own snacks to avoid eating unhealthy, processed snacks you can buy in stores (they will leave you hungry and craving more). I love portioning my homemade hummus in containers and packing it with veggie sticks placed in small baggies so that each day I can just grab and go. This works well with any of my snacks on page x.

- Don't get bored! A downside of meal prep is the meals can sometimes begin to taste the same. You can only have chicken and rice so many times before the thought of it alone causes unquenchable rage. To prevent this, I cook half of my main protein (chicken in this instance, or plant-based proteins) with different spices than the other half. For instance, I make one half of my chicken Italian flavored, perked up with herbs and garlic powder. The other half is made with Indian spices such as cumin and curry powder. Choose whichever combinations of spices you like most and run with it. Small changes go a long way toward making meal prepping both enjoyable and sustainable.

- The meal prep sequence in my 28-day meal plan shows you how to prep by recipe. I find that this is the best method when you are following specific recipes throughout the week, as you'll do on my plan. Sometimes I might multitask by chopping ingredients for one recipe while another one is baking.

BUDGET SAVER TIP #4:
GRADUATE TO PLANT-BASED PROTEINS

With the ever-increasing prices of meat products and worries over how meat is produced, it might be time to start adding more plant-based proteins to your diet. Some of the best (and the cheapest) are:

- Beans—perfect in soups, salads, burritos, and veggie burgers
- Hemp seeds—an ingredient rich in omega-6 and omega-3 fats

- Lentils—delicious in stews and Indian dishes such as daal
- Quinoa—a high-protein alternative to rice or pasta
- Seitan—a great substitute for fish, beef, and soy. This protein isn't covered in detail in this book but can be a great substitute.
- Spirulina—perfect for smoothies
- Tempeh—a fermented soybean-based food that subs for animal protein in many dishes
- Fermented Tofu—a soybean-based food that subs for animal protein in many dishes

Traveling with Your Prepped Meals

I do a lot of traveling, which can mean encountering a lot of rich, fattening foods (as well as meals that seem healthy but aren't) everywhere from airports to gas stations to restaurants. To avoid them, I travel with prepped meals. Here's what I've found works best:

- Book a hotel room with a mini-fridge and head to the nearest grocery store. You can then store delicious and healthy options in the mini-fridge, like Greek yogurt (if you eat dairy; otherwise, opt for a soy-based yogurt or coconut yogurt) or hummus, so that you don't indulge too much while away from home. Also, stock on up healthy snacks, like kale chips, raw almonds, and fruit, while you're there.
- When meal prepping on the go, locate a grocery store such as Whole Foods that has a large salad bar. You can put various ingredients in small containers and refrigerate them for your meals.
- Portion out oatmeal in a container and pack it in your bag. If you want to eat oatmeal on an airplane, ask for hot water. Add a protein boost by mixing in a scoop of protein powder with each portion of oatmeal. You can do the same in your hotel room. I personally use the Just Add Water brand for protein powder, as it's pre-portioned and very convenient to carry with you.

- Follow TSA guidelines for packing food. You may be surprised to find out that items like nut butters and hummus are considered a liquid by TSA. And bring a water bottle with you, but fill it up after you've passed through security. I always carry mint and green tea bags with me to add to my water bottles so that it's more appealing to drink while I fly.

- Bring salads, stir-fries, fruit, vegetables, nuts, and other snacks on your flights. Most people are surprised to find out that you can absolutely bring your own food through security, as long as it's not a liquid. That delicious soup of yours? No go. A mason jar salad with the dressing mixed in? All good! Worth noting is that when arriving in another country, you can't take any fresh produce in, but dried snacks are fine.

- Go with what works. If you're stuck in a situation without many good options, make the best available choice. Of course, fast food isn't ideal. But if you are on a highway in the middle of nowhere, a grilled chicken sandwich or a salad is a far better choice than a burger and fries, even if neither option is as ideal as your normal prepped food.

Meal Prepping and Restaurants

I know what you're thinking: "Can I eat out at restaurants while following this plan?"

Yes, and you know what? You can prep at those restaurants. Remember, the more closely you follow the four-week plan, the better results you'll see. Still, I want you to walk away from reading this book and following this plan with a renewed sense of control over your body and your food choices, even after the 28 days are over—and that means learning how to make the best choices while eating out!

So you'll want to choose places that have healthy selections on their menus, such as veggie plates, grilled chicken or fish, and lots of salad choices. Check the menu closely too, looking for menu options that say "steamed," "roasted," "baked," or "grilled"; avoid anything fried.

Don't be too shy about asking for modifications. I don't hesitate to ask if a dish can be cooked differently. For example, I ask the chef to leave off the cheese or prepare the dish with less salt, or I ask for half the rice (especially with sushi). If all else fails, I inform the waitstaff that I'm vegan. They're usually glad to show me the healthiest plant-based options or will create something if they don't have it on the menu.

If I go out to eat at a not-so-healthy place, I share dishes with my friends. I love Italian food, for example, particularly fresh pasta. Rather than feel guilty about eating it, I split it with a friend. Plus, I always order a side of steamed veggies for the entire table. We eat it first, like an appetizer, and this fills us up so we're not ravenous by the time the entrees arrive.

Here's the beauty of eating out: Restaurants typically serve big portions—which is bad for dieters but great for dieting meal preppers. You can box up what you don't eat, and voilà, you have prepped food for the next few days. So ask for a to-go box, one of the meal prepper's best friends.

I normally advise against hitting all-you-can-eat buffets or establishments that have huge portions for little money, because the food may be bad quality and laced with hidden sugar and salt. However, many of these places serve steamed foods, such as shrimp or crab legs, steamed veggies, and fresh fruit. Load up your plate; what you don't eat goes right into those to-go boxes.

Serve Up Success

If you've never meal prepped before, take it slow. Start with the tips I give initially and get comfortable in the kitchen. Then, once you've mastered your first Sunday prep session, try out week one and see how it goes. If everything worked well and you feel great, progress to week two. Keep going from there. The more you meal prep, the easier it becomes and the more you'll enjoy cooking new recipes.

If, along the way, you find that there are too many recipes in each week's plan, choose the ones you like best and prep only those for the week. There is no right or wrong way to meal prep. I definitely don't want you to feel so overwhelmed that you don't do any of it.

Like so many things in life, meal prep is all about making small but permanent changes. Little changes can impact your life in big ways. Choosing to meal prep means you are choosing a healthier and happier lifestyle. You are shunning the fast foods, processed foods, and junk foods that we all turn to because of our busy schedules. Nothing comes easy, but if you focus on meal prep, you will love the results.

Now, before you hit your kitchen, I want to tell you about some amazing ingredients that you will use over the course of your four-week plan. These items will take your health to new heights and will help you drop pounds. That's where we're going in Part Two of this book.

Part Two

Super Prep

CHAPTER 4
Super Meals

My meal prep weight-loss solution involves something other plans don't emphasize: fortifying your meals with "superfoods" and prepping what I call "super meals."

You've probably heard about superfoods, but you may not know exactly what they are. And you've likely heard that certain foods will increase your energy and deliver health benefits of one kind or another. Case in point: the last time you ate a goji berry—a superfood—did you feel younger and have more energy? Probably not. Let me explain.

I discovered superfoods after moving back to London in 2012, when I was slowly finding my way toward health. I went into Whole Foods, looking for some new foods that could aid in my transition to a better lifestyle. I picked up small bags of spirulina, turmeric, maca powder, chia seeds, bee pollen, and a few other ingredients I had never heard of before. The labels on the bags described the benefits of each ingredient and how they could vastly improve my health. Naturally, I was sold. I desperately wanted to feel better and would try anything.

About $100 later, with around seven items in my basket, I went home and realized I had spent a lot of money on ingredients I knew nothing about and didn't know how to use. It's not like I was making good money at the time either. I was living on a minimal income from modeling, so $100 was a lot of money. It still is today.

I tried each of these superfoods on their own and was underwhelmed. No one can eat chia seeds all day and expect to be a pleasant person. Turmeric made its way into my stir-fry, though it was not something I wanted to eat again. At breakfast, I stirred a tablespoon of spirulina into water, drank it down, and nearly threw up. If you laughed at this last sentence, then my guess is you've had a similar experience.

To me, these superfoods were bad-tasting foods, and they lingered in my pantry for quite some time. Yep, what a great way to spend a hundred bucks.

Soon I began taking courses in nutrition, and I obtained a certification in raw foods from the Institute of Optimum Nutrition in London. The more I learned, the more I researched these so-called superfoods and how to use them. I began experimenting with adding them into smoothies. That not-so-pleasant tasting spirulina was actually bearable when combined with delicious fruits and vegetables in my smoothie! Chia seeds were more delicious when made into puddings with coconut milk. Bee pollen and goji berries suddenly became tasty toppings that added pizazz to dishes, such as my overnight oats. Voilà—I fell in love with my concoctions. The more I used these ingredients with other foods, the better I felt.

As I became more educated in health and nutrition and slowly started changing my diet, I binged less frequently, and I actually started craving green smoothies and unprocessed foods. These superfoods had made a difference, and I was feeling better than ever.

I was still concerned, though, that these ingredients were being marketed as a be-all and end-all solution to getting healthy. People were spending tons of money on them without actually seeing much benefit.

Once I began health coaching, I told my clients that if they weren't already eating a healthy diet, these superfoods weren't going to have much of an effect. You have to start with the best ingredients from the grocery store, including fruits, vegetables, legumes, grains, nuts, seeds, eggs, and so forth, and prep them. Then you can add in those supplemental superfoods.

When you do that, you create a delicious meal that is loaded with all sorts of healthful nutrients. Take kale, for example. When you pair this super vegetable with beets, another super vegetable; chia seeds, a super ingredient; quinoa, a super grain; and top it off with cilantro, a super herb, and a dressing made with lemon, a super fruit, and turmeric, a super spice, you have one hell of a *super meal.*

As a result of my work in nutrition and cooking, I developed my own classifications of superfoods:

Super ingredients	Super grains
Super vegetables	Super herbs and spices
Super fruits	Super beverages

And so I began emphasizing the importance of prepping super meals—a delicious combination of all of these categories of superfoods, fortified with one or more super ingredients. I found that eating super meals had benefits such as reduced bloating, increased weight loss, more energy, clearer skin, and fewer cravings. By prepping and eating super meals, you don't need to count calories, and you won't need to keep dieting.

This is how I've been eating for years, and trust me, it works. Check out my Instagram feed to see photos of super meals, and the results that these meals yield. I am stronger than I've ever been, I have higher endurance, and I sleep better. I no longer crave coffee. My skin is finally clear, after years of battling skin problems. And yes, I have a body of which I'm proud.

In this book, I've created delicious cooking methods and recipes that integrate super ingredients and superfoods right into your meals—no popping supplements or mixing powders in water or juice. Throughout the book, you'll learn how to combine them into your prepped meals in order to boost your nutrition.

In the next six chapters, we will dive into each of these categories with explanations of why these ingredients are good for you and how best to eat them. Sorry, fast-food joints, but there is a new super meal in town, and it's not going to make you feel like crap; quite the opposite, in fact.

BUDGET SAVER
TIP #5: SHOP AROUND

Shopping is a part of prepping. Of course, shopping around and comparing prices can be extremely time-consuming, but the savings are impressive. Simply going to your local farmer's market to purchase your veggies can cut a considerable amount off your total food bill, and the produce will probably be organic. Look for special promotions at your supermarket too.

If you have access to Asian or ethnic markets, you'll find good deals. Nuts, spices, and vegetables, for example, are sometimes half the price of those sold in conventional supermarkets. Check out the international aisles in grocery stores too—many times you'll find cheaper prices on foods that sell at a higher cost in the regular aisles.

If you find that you are very low on time, then I recommend delivery services, like Amazon, which can drop off everything you need right at your door. This has been a lifesaver for me in busy periods because it's there when I arrive home and all I have to do is prep, no shopping required.

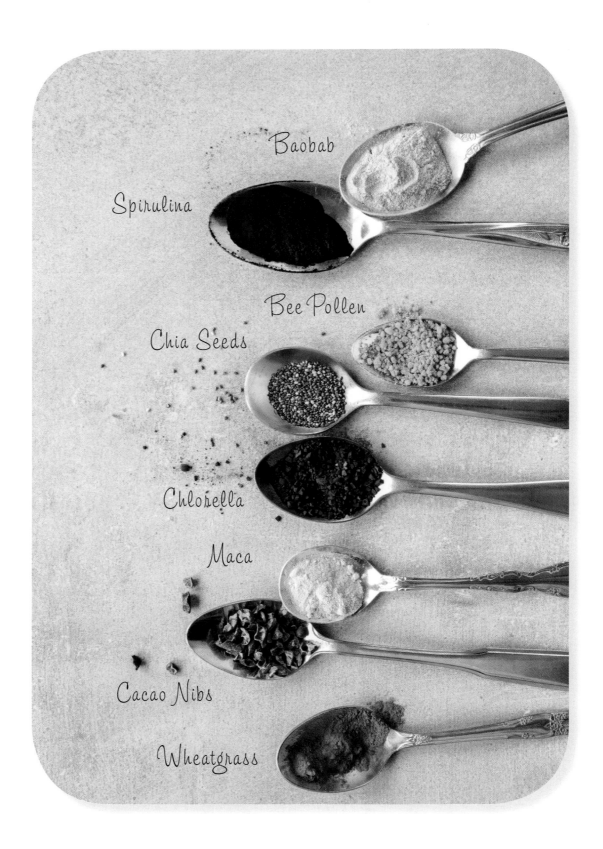

Baobab

Spirulina

Bee Pollen

Chia Seeds

Chlorella

Maca

Cacao Nibs

Wheatgrass

CHAPTER 5

Super Ingredients

I love to add super ingredients to my meals, so let's take a look at my favorites and what they can do for you. Don't worry; it's not necessary to go out and buy every single ingredient below. Start with one or two, use them in various recipes, then gradually add more to your pantry. If I had to recommend a few right off the bat, I suggest spirulina, maca powder, and chia seeds.

Here's a rundown of all the ingredients and how to use them.

Baobab

What is it? Baobab is a fruit that comes from a tree of the same name. The tree grows wild in Africa and Madagascar and has been widely introduced elsewhere. The fruit is available in powder form.

How does it help? The baobab fruit is said to have three times as much vitamin C as an orange, contain 50 percent more calcium than spinach, and be a good source of antioxidants. A 2014 study published in the *Journal of Ethnopharmacology* suggested that increasing your intake of baobab and other African herbs may be useful in preventing or reducing the progression of lifestyle-related diseases, such as heart disease and type 2 diabetes.

How much do you need? One to two teaspoons daily.

How to take it? Mix it into smoothies or herbal tea.

Bee Pollen

What is it? Bee pollen is collected and processed from plants as the insects carry out their job of pollinating plants and flowers.

How does it help? Bee pollen is one of the richest sources of vitamins in a single food. It helps with endurance, strength, speed, and recovery from exercise. A 2016 review article published in the *Journal of the Science of Food and Agriculture* reported that it can also reduce allergies and hay fever, help control cravings, and improve circulation.

How much do I need? One teaspoon a day.

How do I take it? Sprinkle bee pollen on oats in the morning, put in a smoothie, or mix it into bliss balls, such as my Coconut Dreamsicle Bliss Balls, by adding 1 teaspoon into the mixture before you roll them. You can also eat it directly; let it dissolve on your tongue for an instant energy hit.

Cacao

What is it? Cacao is unheated cocoa powder. Both cacao and cocoa come from the cacao bean, which is the source of chocolate, but cacao is raw and unprocessed, and therefore more nutritious.

How does it help? Raw cacao contains the highest magnesium levels of any food. Because of the magnesium, cacao helps promote relaxation, reduce stress, suppress appetite for better weight management, and control blood sugar. It also boosts immune health due to its high content of zinc, iron, and vitamin C. These health benefits are largely due to cacao's high antioxidant and phytochemical content, according to a 2015 review article published in *Current Pharmaceutical Biotechnology*.

How much do I need? One to three teaspoons a day.

How do I take it? Mix it into smoothies, create hot chocolate, add it to bliss balls, use it in stir-fry sauces, flavor cakes with it, or make my Chocolate Orange Smoothie (page 163).

Chia Seeds

What are they? Chia seeds are a relative of mint and are native to Mexico and Guatemala. Although they date back to the time of the Aztecs as an important food crop, they didn't become popular in North America until about thirty years ago.

How do they help? Chia seeds are high in the minerals magnesium, calcium, iron, and zinc, which play a role in energy creation, strong bones, and immunity. These mighty little seeds are also a plant source of omega-3 fats, which reduce inflammation in the body, promote clear skin, and lower LDL ("bad") cholesterol, while raising levels of HDL ("good") cholesterol. Chia assists with weight loss because the seeds are high in fiber and expand slightly in the stomach, helping you feel full. Several journals in recent years, including the *Journal of Biomedicine and Biotechnology*, *Nutricion Hospitalaria,* and *Advances in Food and Nutrition Research,* have enumerated in detail the health attributes of this potent little seed.

How much do I need? One to two tablespoons daily.

How do I take it? Make chia seed pudding, sprinkle them on oats, add them to smoothies, scatter them over salads, or use them as an egg replacement in baking.

Chlorella

What is it? Chlorella is a form of pure green algae that has existed naturally on earth for thousands of years.

How does it help? This algae promotes a healthy immune system, detoxes the liver, helps with digestion, and promotes cellular rejuvenation. Because of all these qualities, researchers writing in a 2016 issue of *Current Pharmaceutical Design* call chlorella "a multifunctional dietary supplement."

How much do I need? One to two teaspoons daily.

How do I take it? Add it to stews, cakes, Bliss Balls, smoothies, and juices. While it's not included in any specific recipes in this book, it's a great ingredient to add and I carry it everywhere when traveling.

Maca Powder

What is it? Maca is a member of the radish family. Its primary usable part is its potato-like tuberous root. It is usually sold as a nutty powder, but it also comes in capsules.

How does it help? Highly nutritious, the plant contains about 13 percent protein, is rich in vitamins and minerals, and is an adaptogen (a substance that helps the body resist stress). Maca is also purported to enhance libido and sexual performance, according to a 2015 report published in the *Journal of Sexual Medicine*.

How much do you need? One tablespoon daily.

How to take it? You can bake with maca powder, use it in smoothies, or—my personal favorite—blend it into coffee.

Spirulina

What is it? Spirulina is a genus of blue-green algae used as a nutritional supplement.

How does it help? An overview of spirulina, published in a 2013 article in *Mini Reviews in Medicinal Chemistry,* noted that this algae is brimming with nutrients, including B vitamins, beta-carotene, gamma-linolenic acid (a good fatty acid), iron, calcium, magnesium, manganese, potassium, selenium, zinc, and bioflavonoids. One notable benefit is that spirulina is about 65 percent protein. Its proteins are "complete," meaning that they have all eight essential amino acids, plus some nonessential ones. In that regard, spirulina is similar to animal protein, but without the artery-clogging fats, or the hormones or antibiotics that are in some meats.

How much do you need? One to two teaspoons a day.

How to take it? There are many ways to use spirulina: in smoothies and fresh-squeezed juices; sprinkled on popcorn, with other seasonings; in dips and salsas; and in raw chocolate desserts.

Wheatgrass

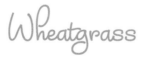

What is it? Wheatgrass is the young grass of the wheat plant, *Triticum aestivum.*

How does it help? Wheatgrass is a great way to pump up your veggie intake. It delivers such a nutrient punch that one ounce of it is rumored to be the equivalent of more than two pounds of fresh fruit and vegetables in terms of vitamins, minerals, trace elements, and phytonutrients. It has been shown to possess anti-cancer, anti-ulcer, antioxidant, and anti-arthritic activity due to the presence of many biologically active compounds and minerals, according to a 2015 analysis reported in the *Journal of Pharmacy and Bioallied Sciences.*

How much do you need? 1 teaspoon daily.

How to take it? You can add it to smoothies, soups, and juices.

There you have it—super ingredients for super health as you lose weight. Stock up on these ingredients, and you will supercharge your meals, your nutrition, and your well-being. Remember, though, that when eaten alone these ingredients aren't always the best. That's why, in the next few chapters, I show you how to pair ingredients for optimal results.

CHAPTER 6

Super Vegetables

Let me first say that all vegetables are super vegetables. They contain a wide range of nutrients, including potassium, fiber, folate, vitamins A, E, and C, and phytochemicals (non-vitamin nutrients that have disease-preventing powers) that help your body thrive and stay healthy. Try to eat as many different-colored vegetables as possible. Orange vegetables, like carrots and sweet potatoes, have generous amounts of vitamin A, for instance. And green vegetables, such as kale and spinach, are chock full of iron and calcium.

If you don't care for veggies, I'll make you a bet: you will like them after you try the recipes in this book. You might even love them. I've turned many a vegetable hater into a vegetable lover with my plant-based cooking. Just give the recipes an honest try. I'm sure they will end your "I don't like vegetables" mindset.

Here are the vegetables you'll be prepping and cooking during the next four weeks. Enjoy!

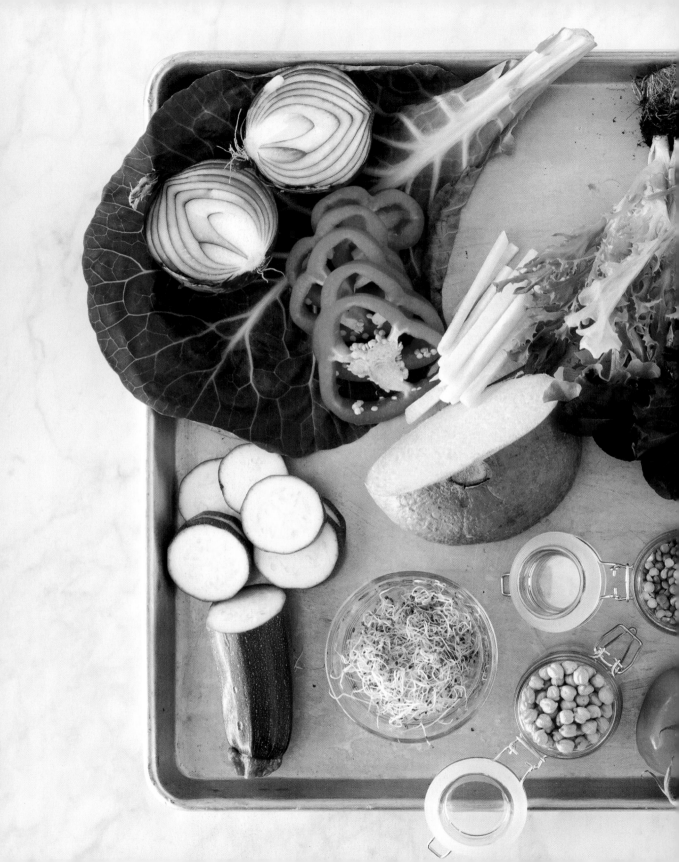

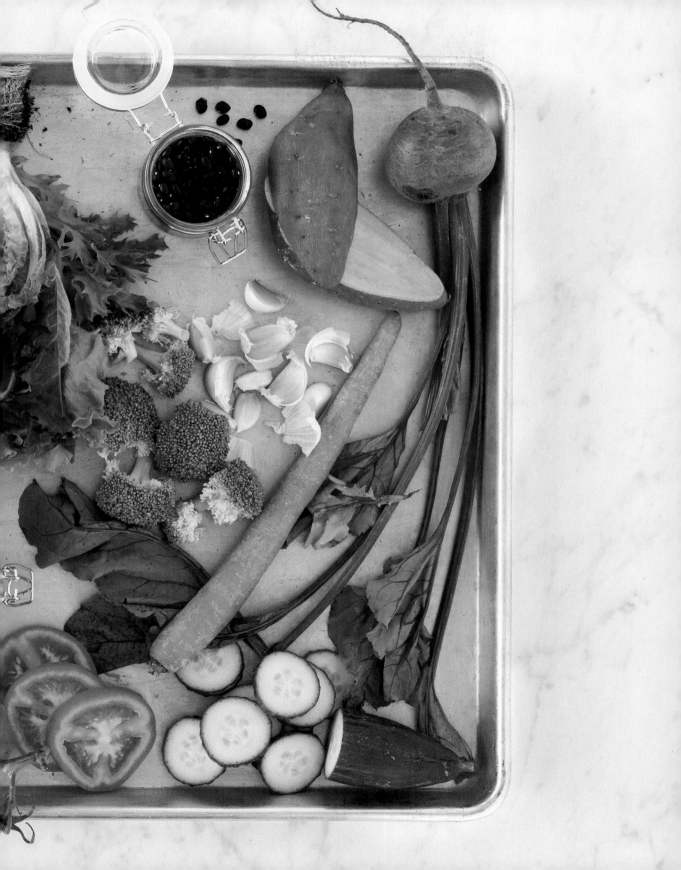

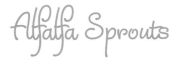

Alfalfa Sprouts

What are they? Alfalfa sprouts are the shoots of the alfalfa plant, harvested before they become a full-grown plant. Because they are so small, the sprouts contain a concentrated amount of many vitamins and minerals such as calcium, vitamin K, and vitamin C. Alfalfa sprouts are also very low in calories, with just 8 calories a cup.

How do they help? Alfalfa sprouts contain very powerful antioxidants, reported a 2016 study published in *Regulatory Toxicology and Pharmacology*. They're also high in saponin, a phytochemical that binds with bile acids and cholesterol, washing these fatty compounds from the body. Alfalfa sprouts are loaded with folate, a B vitamin that protects the heart and brain and guards against birth defects.

Always eaten raw, these sprouts infuse your body with their life energy, enzymes, and vitality, according to raw food advocates. I think sprouts are among the best raw veggies you can eat.

How to use them? Alfalfa sprouts are delicious in salads, sandwiches, and wraps.

Beans

What are they? "Beans" is the collective name for the large seeds of several types of plant families. Some of the most popular bean varieties include lima, black, black-eyed pea, red kidney, chickpea (also called garbanzo), navy, pinto, and edamame (a form of soybeans).

How do they help? I consider beans a super vegetable because they contain a hefty nutrient package. They are an excellent source of plant protein and cholesterol-lowering fiber, and they provide important nutrients such as calcium, iron, folic acid, and potassium. Including beans as a regular part of a healthy diet may help prevent and control diabetes and help reduce the risk of high blood pressure and stroke. Also, one serving of beans (about ½ cup) provides 20 percent or more of your daily fiber needs.

How to use them? You can eat them as a main or side dish; turn them into veggie burgers; use them in soups, stews, and chilis; fold them into tacos or burritos; toss them in salads; and substitute them for flour in brownies and cookies (black beans are particularly useful in baked goods). Ways to use beans are virtually limitless.

Beets

What are they? Beets are a root veggie that have been enjoyed since ancient times. The Romans were among the first to recognize the nutritional superpowers of the beet, and in the Middle Ages physicians used beets to treat digestive and blood-related illnesses.

How do they help? Beets are endowed with a pigment called betacyanin that gives them their bright red color. This pigment also has anti-inflammatory and cancer-preventing benefits, reports a 2017 review published in *Phytotherapy Research*. Beets are packed with potassium, vitamin C, and folate.

How to use them? Beets can be baked, boiled, or steamed. Enjoy them as simple side dishes, in salads, and in soups. I love to turn them into hummus.

Bell Peppers

What are they? Bell peppers have been with us for thousands of years, originally cultivated in South and Central America before being introduced to Europe by Christopher Columbus. They are now grown throughout the world, but mainly in China, Mexico, and the United States.

How do they help? Bell peppers contain more than thirty different carotenoids, which are a type of phytochemical with antioxidant powers. This nutritional combo, along with their high levels of folate, vitamin A, dietary fiber, vitamin E, and vitamin B$_6$, make bell peppers one of the most effective weapons against cancer, heart disease, eye disorders, and diabetes. Bell peppers supply more than twice the vitamin C found in oranges.

How to use them? You can eat them raw, roasted, or sautéed. They're delicious in salads, soups, chili, and many other dishes. You can also stuff bell peppers for a flavorful entrée.

Broccoli

What is it? Broccoli is a member of the cabbage family and is considered one of the healthiest vegetables you can eat.

How does it help? This green vegetable is regarded by many as the single best cancer-preventive substance in the produce bin. Broccoli takes center stage as the healthiest of the cruciferous vegetables, a group of super vegetables to which cauliflower, Brussels sprouts, and cabbage belong. Broccoli is packed with B vitamins, vitamin C, and folate, along with the carotenoids beta-carotene and lutein; lutein is potent at averting degenerative eye disorders such as cataracts and age-related macular degeneration.

How to use it? Enjoy it raw or cooked in just about anything: salads, soups, or side dishes. Or use it to scoop up hummus or another dip. Raw broccoli is higher in vitamin C, but cooking makes the vegetable's carotenoids more bioavailable to the body.

Carrots

What are they? Carrots are a root vegetable, usually colored orange, although there are white, purple, black, red, white, and yellow varieties too.

How do they help? Carrots are best known as an abundant source of provitamin A (which can be converted to active vitamin A) and beta-carotene, a carotenoid. Carotenoids are potent nutrients that protect cells and tissues from damage from free radicals, enhance immunity, protect against sunburn reactions, and help delay the onset of certain types of cancer, according to a 2016 article published in *Sub-Cellular Biochemistry*.

How to use them? Enjoy raw carrots grated or sliced into most any dish, from salads and stir-fries to stews and baked goods. Snacking on raw carrots will curb hunger in no time. They are also heavenly when roasted with olive oil and salt or cooked and pureed as a soup.

Cauliflower

What is it? Like broccoli, cauliflower is one of the healthiest veggies on the planet.

How does it help? Cauliflower might seem boring and bland, though it is anything but when it comes to nutrition. It is loaded with nutrients that fight inflammation, such as vitamin C. Cauliflower is also abundant in thiamin, riboflavin, niacin, magnesium, phosphorus, fiber, vitamin B_6, folate, pantothenic acid, potassium, and manganese. My favorite benefit of cauliflower is that it helps detoxify in a couple of ways: it contains detoxifying antioxidants as well as natural substances called glucosinolates that activate detoxification enzymes—a fact that has been reported in several scientific reviews. This nutritionally powerful vegetable may provide substantial protection against cardiovascular disease, cancer, diabetes, and rheumatoid arthritis.

How to use it? A newly popular way to prep cauliflower is as "rice," in which you grate it, then boil it. As such, it forms a low-carb rice-like granule that can replace rice in many recipes (I like to use it in homemade sushi). Cauliflower is delicious raw, roasted, or sautéed. You can make a mock mashed potato dish by cooking it until tender and mashing it with garlic, coconut oil, salt, and pepper.

Celery

What is it? Celery, which has been around since antiquity, is what we think of as "rabbit food" when we diet—something boring and unsatisfying. But when you prepare this stalky vegetable properly, it brings a lot of zest and flavor to foods.

How does it help? Celery is high in fiber, which moves food through the digestive tract more quickly, and therefore helps lower your risk for digestive diseases. Like most green veggies, it's full of vitamins and minerals: vitamin A and folate, vitamin K, several B vitamins, potassium, manganese, copper, phosphorus, magnesium, and calcium. There is a high concentration of flavonoids in celery too. One of these is apigen, which appears to help prevent cancers of the gastrointestinal tract, reports a 2017 article in *Expert Opinion on Drug Metabolism and Toxicology*.

How to use it? Celery makes a terrific crunchy snack. I like to use it in salads, soups, stews, and stuffings. If you like to juice, celery (and its leaves) make a great addition to fresh juice because of its high water content and its flavor profile, and it is great in smoothies, as it is very refreshing. Just make sure to chop it up first for both juices and smoothies.

Cucumber

What is it? The cucumber is a member of the gourd family, and it grows on a vine. In some circles, it is considered a fruit, but in the culinary world, it is a veggie.

How does it help? Like most veggies, cucumbers are packed with vitamins and minerals. But they have some lesser-known nutritional qualities. For example, cukes contain an anti-inflammatory flavonoid called fisetin that guards brain health and protects against cancer, reported a 2013 study in *Antioxidants and Redox Signalling.* Cucumbers are 95 percent water, making them a great veggie for cleansing and detoxing.

How to use it? My favorite way to enjoy cucumbers is to slice them up and dip them in hummus. Of course, cucumbers are wonderful on salads and in sandwiches too. You can also juice with them, thanks to their high water content.

Garlic

What is it? Garlic comes in a bulb, which is composed of many individual cloves. Just about everyone knows that garlic packs a very strong scent. It is a wonderful addition to many dishes.

How does it help? Garlic is one of the best detoxifiers you can eat, indisputable as a cleansing food. Studies show that the long-term use of garlic protects the arteries against plaque buildup and works to lower abnormally elevated cholesterol. It also has antimicrobial activity, assisting in maintaining good bacteria (probiotics) in the gut. While I personally love the taste of garlic, you can also take it in supplement form to receive many of its benefits without the smell or taste.

How to use it? Garlic can be used in salad dressings and marinades, on roasted vegetables and any type of meat, poultry, or fish, and in Italian, Mexican, Greek, and Asian dishes, among others. There are few foods you can't use it on, except for maybe ice cream!

Green Leafy Vegetables

What are they? Here I'm talking about kale, spinach, collard greens, lettuce, and other leafy veggies.

How do they help? This group of veggies seems to have it all: phytochemicals, vitamins, and minerals. They are thus protective against many life-threatening diseases. Because of this nutritional bounty, the U.S. Department of Agriculture recommends incorporating at least 3 cups (cooked, or 6 cups raw) in your diet every week. Greens have big nutritional perks such as vitamins A, C, K, and folate. Many varieties of these vegetables supply 20 to 30 percent of your daily recommendation for calcium in a 1-cup cooked serving.

How to use them? These delicious, protective plants are so versatile. Use them raw in salads, sandwiches, wraps, and smoothies, or cooked as side dishes, in soups or stews, even as toppings for pizza.

Jicama

What is it? Jicama is a root vegetable. I have heard it described as "the best veggie you're not eating" because it is so nutritious, low in calories, and versatile. It looks like a cross between an apple and a turnip.

How does it help? What distinguishes jicama from many vegetables is that it contains a "prebiotic," a beneficial fiber that feeds probiotics, the friendly bacteria in the gut. It has a low glycemic index too, and therefore is helpful in controlling blood sugar. High in vitamin C, it also supports immune function.

How to use it? You can eat this nutritional superstar raw, sliced into salads, or sautéed in stir-fries.

Lentils

What are they? Lentils are legumes, just like other types of beans. They grow in pods that contain either one or two lentil seeds that are round and are oftentimes smaller than the tip of a pencil eraser.

How do they help? Lentils are among the healthiest legumes you can eat, and they deserve more attention in our diets. First, they're an excellent source of fiber. They are of special benefit in controlling diabetes because their high fiber content halts blood sugar from rising too quickly after a meal. Lentils have more to offer too. They supply many vital minerals, several key B vitamins, and protein—all with virtually no unhealthy fat. The caloric price tag of all this nutrition? Just 115 calories for ½ cup cooked lentils. Lentils fill you up—not out. Want to keep your body fit and happy? Eat lentils.

How to use them? I cook frequently with lentils. Compared to other types of dried beans, lentils are quick cookers and easy to prep. They readily absorb a variety of wonderful flavors from other foods, herbs, and spices with which they are paired. I use them in soups, stews, and salads, and as side dishes.

Onion

What is it? I think everyone knows what an onion is—the popular veggie that makes your eyes water when you prep it. When you slice an onion, you break cells, releasing a compound that causes you to tear up. If you refrigerate an onion prior to prepping it, it is less likely to make you cry.

How does it help? I realize many people avoid onions because of what they do to your breath. But this vegetable contains a lot of miracle nutrients, including sulfur, responsible for lowering blood pressure and discouraging tumor growth; quercetin, a flavonoid with potent antioxidant activity; and saponins, which help fight high cholesterol and tumor formation. A 2015 review published in *Critical Reviews in Food Science and Nutrition* noted that the compounds in onions have a range of health benefits, including anti-cancer properties, anti-blood-clotting activity, anti-asthma benefits, and antibiotic effects.

How to use it? There are very few dishes in which onions cannot be used. They're great in salads, on sandwiches, and in all sorts of ethnic dishes. The list is virtually endless.

Sweet Potatoes

What are they? Despite the name, sweet potatoes aren't in the same family as potatoes. Instead, they are a tuber, which is the stem of a plant, containing high levels of vitamins.

How do they help? Loaded with vitamin C, potassium, and fiber, they are exceptional sources of beta-carotene (which gives them their orange hue) and vitamin A. Both nutrients may protect against some cancers, loss of vision from age-related macular degeneration, and heart disease. Unlike white potatoes, sweet potatoes score low on the glycemic index. This means that when you eat one, your blood sugar rises only half as high as it might after eating a white potato. So basically, sweet potatoes can help maintain steady blood sugar and ease cravings.

How to use them? Sweet potatoes are best baked and eaten as a side dish. You can also use the flesh to make pies and other desserts. I like to stuff them, as I do in my Loaded Mexican Baked Sweet Potato (page 203). Keep them in a dry, cool place like your pantry, and they'll stay good for a month; at room temperature, they'll go bad after a week. Don't refrigerate your sweet potatoes either, or else they'll absorb flavors from other foods, and their starch content will increase.

Tomatoes

What are they? There's an ongoing discussion as to whether tomatoes should be classified as a fruit or a vegetable (they have the botanical qualities of fruits but are enjoyed as veggies).

How do they help? Tomatoes win nutritional points by delivering hefty amounts of fiber, B vitamins, vitamin C, iron, and potassium. They're also the single highest source of the antioxidant lycopene—a plant pigment that may even be more powerful than beta-carotene when it comes to battling the destructive effects of health-stealing free radicals. Unchecked free radical activity has been linked to cancer, heart disease, and illnesses associated with the aging process. Cooked tomatoes and tomato products—sauce, juice, and puree—have two to eight times as much available lycopene as when eaten raw. And there's solid clinical proof that tomato eaters have lower incidences of digestive tract malignancies and prostate cancer.

How to use them? Tomatoes are perfect for salads, soups, juices, side dishes, snacks, pizzas, and so many other things. You can stuff them, use them in practically all ethnic cuisines, and more. They add a beautiful color and an abundance of nutrients to any dish.

Zucchini

What is it? Zucchini actually sits under the umbrella of summer squash, which refers to squashes that get harvested before their rinds harden, unlike, say, pumpkins and butternut squash. Here is another one of those plant foods that is technically a fruit, because it comes from a flower. Zucchini is so popular that there is even a National Zucchini Day, celebrated on August 8.

How does it help? Nutritionally, zucchini delivers potassium that helps reduce blood pressure. Its considerable amount of magnesium helps in keeping blood pressure at a normal level too, and the heart beating at a steady rhythm. Like the cucumber (to which it is related), zucchini keeps the body hydrated with its 95 percent water content. As an excellent source of vitamin C, it is considered a good food for maintaining immune health and fighting respiratory problems. It is also one of the lowest-calorie veggies around: 19 calories per cup of slices.

How to use it? A new popular way to use zucchini is to spiralize it into low-carb noodles that can substitute for pasta. When using zucchini as a replacement to pasta, you can either keep it raw (which I recommend for the health benefits), or boil it in water like normal spaghetti—but for just a few minutes or until soft. The key to raw noodles is mixing your sauce in and allowing it to sit for 20 minutes to become soft. You can also enjoy this low-calorie food in so many different recipes, from bread to soups to lasagna. Of course, you can always grill or roast zucchini with a little olive oil and herbs for a delectable side dish.

My 28-day meal plan takes into consideration all the benefits of these amazing super vegetables. You'll love the way they taste, what they do for your body, and how they make you feel, physically and mentally. Plants rule the world!

CHAPTER 7

Super Fruits

Like vegetables, all fruits are "super." My 28-day plan helps you incorporate a variety of super fruits in your daily diet, including strawberries, blueberries, raspberries, lemons, limes, apples, pineapple, and bananas, along with dried fruits such as dates and goji berries, which have their own unique set of benefits. Fruits are also "nature's candy" and will help you curb cravings for fattening, processed sweets.

Apple

What is it? Apples are grown worldwide and come in so many different varieties, each with a different degree of sweetness.

How does it help? Apples have it all, and that why it's good to eat an apple a day with the skin on. I can't compliment apples enough: they're loaded with fiber, flavonoids, potassium, antioxidants, and vitamins A and C. Apples are a nutritional powerhouse that help every single part of the body stay healthy, from the brain to the heart to the digestive system.

How to use it? The best way to eat an apple is raw—as a delicious, filling, and sweet snack. Like them even sweeter? Then you'll love my Toffee Apples (page 258). Of course, apples are sumptuous when baked, alone or in various fruit-based desserts. They're so sweet when cooked or baked that you hardly need to add sweeteners of any type.

Avocado

What is it? The avocado is actually a fruit, even though we treat it as vegetable, adding it to salads or stuffing it with chicken or tuna salad. It has been with us a long time. Some archaeological evidence shows that avocado consumption goes back almost 10,000 years in central Mexico.

How does it help? The avocado has a very long resume of nutritional benefits: high in fiber, includes most vitamins, and contains several minerals. Compared to most other fruits, avocado is high in fat. But the fat falls into the super-healthy category, because it guards against heart disease. There are also many other health benefits to which the avocado is linked: weight loss, relief of arthritis, lowering of bad cholesterol, skin health, and blood sugar control.

How to use it? Avocado is delicious consumed raw, but it can also be used as the base for guacamole and other dips. Its texture makes it perfect for creating mousse-like desserts and puddings.

Banana

What is it? The banana is a tropical fruit and is considered one of the healthiest fruits on the planet.

How does it help? Bananas are a nutritional gold mine due to the fact

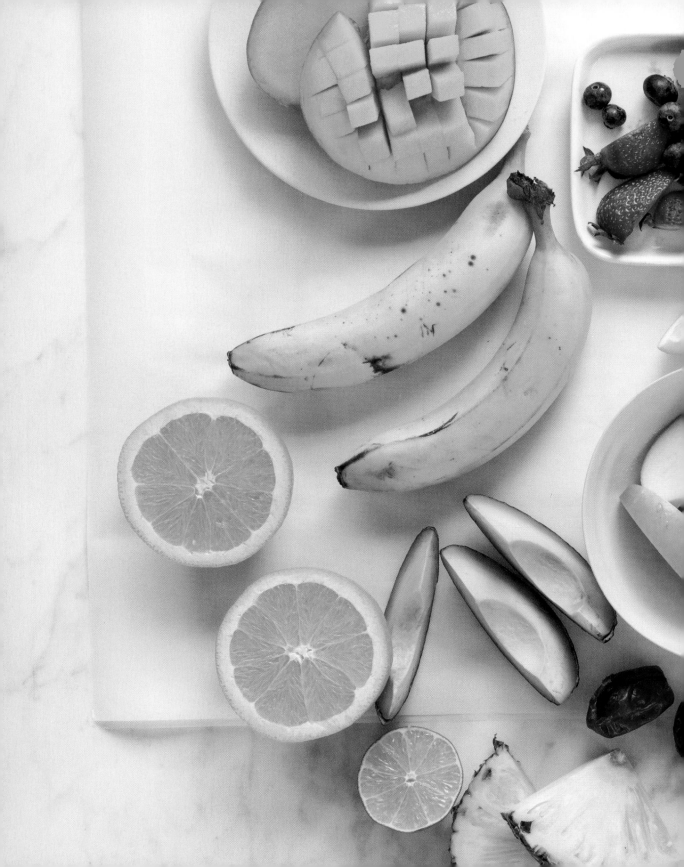

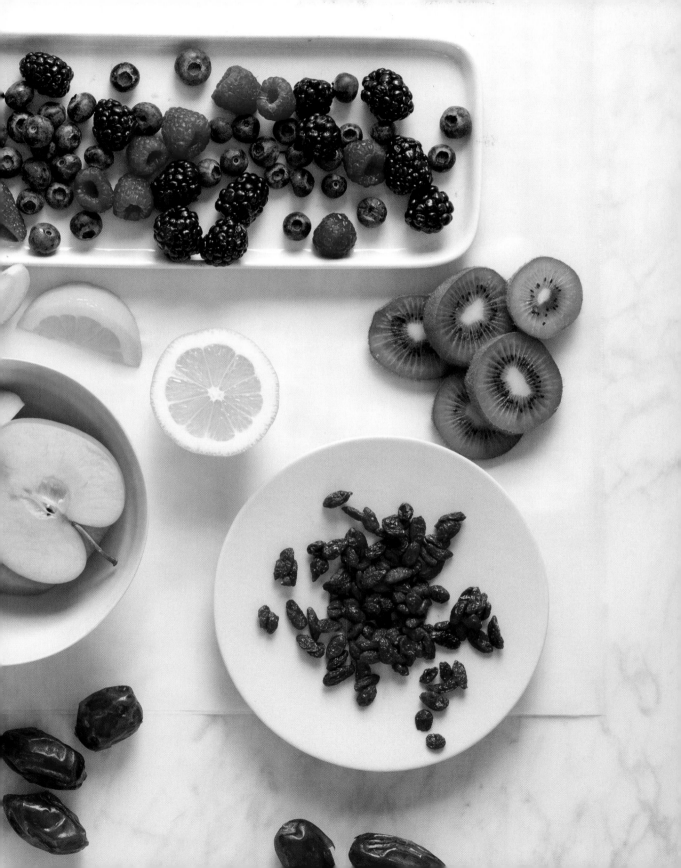

that they contain the mineral potassium, considered essential in regulating blood pressure and promoting heart health. Of course, they're rich in many other nutrients, including magnesium, vitamin B$_6$, and vitamin C—all protectors of heart and brain health.

How to use it? I use bananas mostly in smoothies, or as snacks. I like to freeze bananas, especially as they ripen. I'll slice a banana, wrap up the slices, and place them in the freezer. That way, they're ready to pop in the blender. Another great use is 'nana ice cream, such as my Tropical Treat Ice Cream on page 294.

Berries

What are they? There are many kinds of berries: blueberries, raspberries, strawberries, and others.

How do they help? Sweet and juicy, berries are brimming with valuable phytochemicals, including ellagic acid, which works to shield DNA from cancer-causing agents. Blueberries, in particular, are powerful disease fighters: experiments show that just ⅔ cup yields as much antioxidant power as 1,773 IU of vitamin E or 1,270 milligrams of vitamin C. In addition, all berries are packed with the soluble fiber pectin, which helps curb LDL cholesterol and eases digestion problems. The best part? Berries are low in calories—ranging from about 45 to 80 calories a cup—so you can enjoy their sweetness without worrying about your waistline.

How to use them? I love to have a bowl of berries as a filling, sweet snack. But I also use them in smoothies (usually frozen). Berries make delicious toppings for all sorts of dishes, including cereals. You can also use them in salads as a sweet garnish.

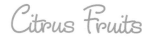

Citrus Fruits

What are they? Grown on flowering trees and shrubs, citrus fruits include oranges, lemons, and limes—all three of which I use throughout this 28-day plan.

How do they help? Citrus fruits are most famous for their high vitamin C content, which boosts immunity and is involved in strengthening collagen, the protein in skin that keeps it firm. They are a great source of fiber too, and have been linked to the prevention of heart disease and cancer, according to a 2017 study published in *Biofactors*.

How to use them? Oranges make wonderful snacks, and sliced, they can serve as a beautiful garnish too (yes, please eat that garnish!). As for lemons and limes, you'll find that I use their juice frequently in recipes, to give dishes a tang and an extra dose of nutrition.

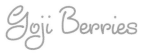

Goji Berries

What are they? Native to China and Tibet, these little fruits have long been used in traditional herbal medicine.

How do they help? High in antioxidants to prevent cell damage and loaded with anti-inflammatory nutrients, these berries protect the brain, eyes, and heart—and may help fight aging, noted a 2008 study published in *Cellular and Molecular Neurobiology*.

How to use them? Add these berries to trail mix, cereals, desserts, bliss balls, oats, smoothies, and salads, or make my Goji Berry Tea (page 113). Have two tablespoons daily to increase your antioxidant intake and for higher energy levels.

Mango

What is it? This tropical fruit has been named the most widely consumed fruit in the world, according to *Medical News Today*. The mango is considered a "drupe": a type of fruit in which an outer fleshy part surrounds a pit with a seed inside. Olives, dates, and coconuts are also types of drupes.

How does it help? Because mangos are rich in a variety of antioxidants, they help fight eye disorders, cancer, asthma, bone weakness, heart disease, and diabetes, to name just a few. Want great hair and skin? Grab a mango. The vitamin A it contains is required for sebum production that keeps your hair moisturized. And its high vitamin C content helps build and maintain collagen.

How to use it? Mango is just so delicious that I like to eat a bowl of it all by itself. You can also use it in fruit salads and smoothies.

Medjool Dates

What are they? Considered the "king of dates," the Medjool variety is larger and softer than most dates—which makes them easier to use in recipes. They originated in the Middle East and North Africa, where they are staples in many dishes.

How do they help? Medjool dates contain skin- and eye-protecting vitamin A and blood-clot-regulating vitamin K. Medjool dates are high in fiber too, and can help combat constipation and other digestive problems. They've also been proven to decrease cholesterol and boost bone health.

How to use them? Medjool dates can serve as a wonderful natural sweetener. You can blend them into smoothies and mix them into desserts, without ever needing to add a grain of sugar. The sticky texture of the dates makes them perfect for binding ingredients together—use them in recipes such as raw bars, sugar-free fudge, and bliss balls.

Pineapple

What is it? Second only to bananas as America's favorite tropical fruit, the pineapple has a spiny outer covering that, when peeled open, yields the juicy, luscious fruit.

How does it help? Like most fruits, the pineapple is vitamin- and antioxidant-rich. Perhaps the most distinguishing nutritional feature of the pineapple is bromelain, an enzyme found in the juice and stem. Bromelain is an anti-inflammatory substance, used to reduce swelling.

How to use it? Pineapple is delicious eaten raw, in fruit salads, and blended into smoothies.

You'll discover some wonderful recipes in the 28-day plan that incorporate these fruits. Or just enjoy them as snacks all on their own.

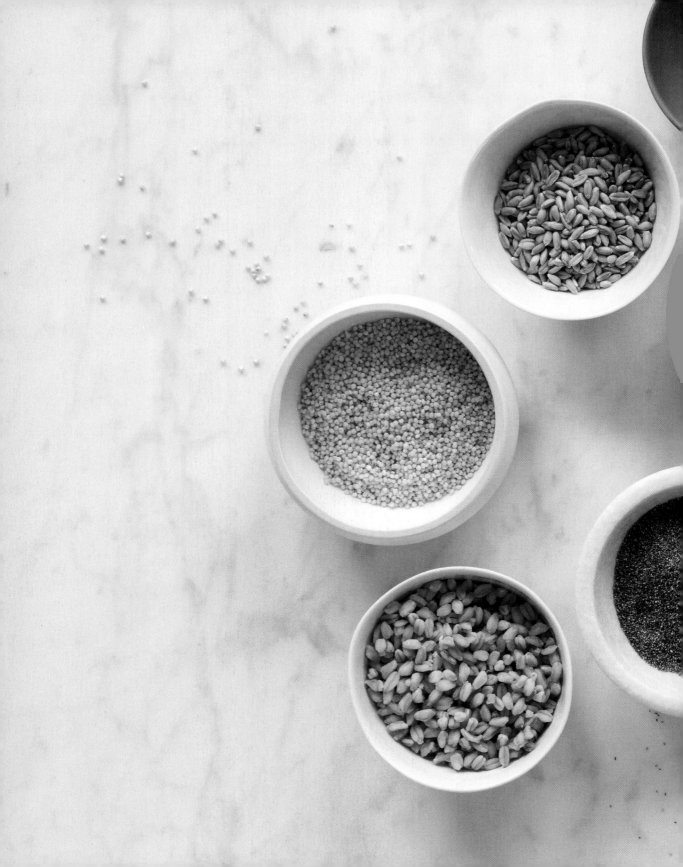

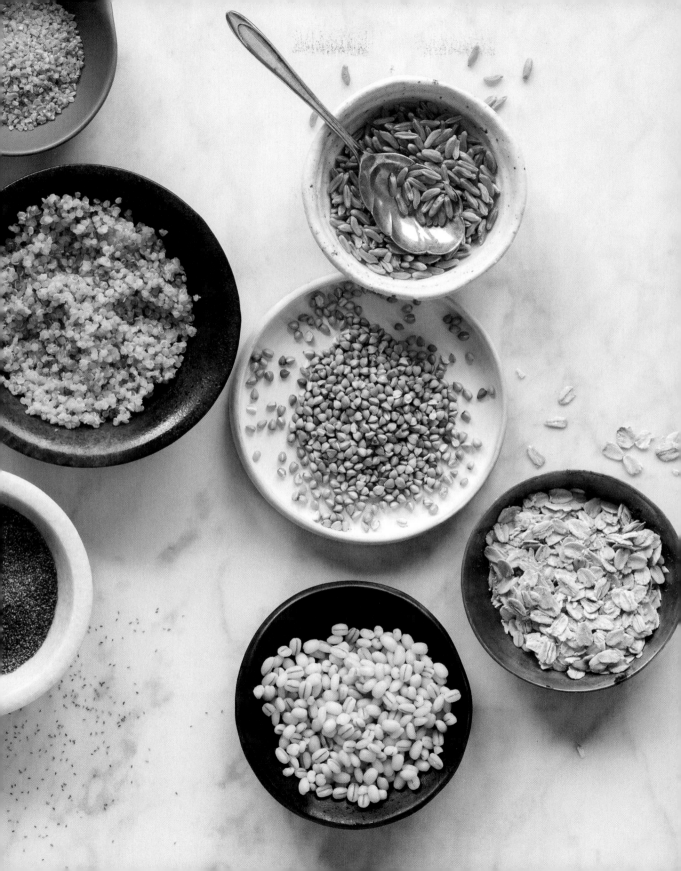

CHAPTER 8

Super Grains

If you haven't met the super grains yet, let me introduce you. All are amazing foods—easy to cook with and delicious. Super grains are chock full of fiber, protein, vitamins, and minerals, along with carbohydrates.

Now don't go carbo-phobic on me and get scared these grains will make you fat. They won't, but I understand where you're coming from. I've been in your shoes. I was once terrified of carbs and wouldn't go near them. But by skipping *good* carbs, my body went into a starvation mode of sorts because I was missing vital proteins and nutrients, and not putting enough energy into my body. This led to bingeing on bad carbs—and gaining weight. Now that I follow a predominantly plant-based diet, I no longer binge on foods that I know won't make me feel good, and I eat as many of these super grains as I want.

Super grains are packed with protein. They supply glucose, the main source of fuel your body runs on, as well as health-protective B vitamins and antioxidants. After adding super grains to my diet, not only did I have more energy throughout the day, but I was sleeping better, and no longer obsessing over my carb intake.

Throughout the recipes in the 28-day plan, I'd like you to mix and match different super grains. If a recipe calls for quinoa but you'd like to try out barley, please do. I promise that you cannot go wrong using any of the below ingredients if you add them to a soup, salad, hot cereal, and so forth. Cooking should be fun, so I do recommend swapping out and experimenting with various ingredients.

Because nutrition, taste, and versatility are a big part of the appeal of my meal prep plan, try to eat a super grain at least once a day.

BUDGET SAVER
TIP #6: SWAP OUT INGREDIENTS

Sometimes simply swapping an ingredient from a recipe can save you several dollars and allows you to adapt a recipe to suit your taste, your time, and what's in your cupboard or fridge! For example, black beans or even quinoa can be used in place of meat in many recipes (like chili or stews). These ingredients are lower in cost, don't have the antibiotics and hormones that meat does, and will leave you feeling incredibly satiated.

Buckwheat Groats

What is it? Trivia question: Is buckwheat a member of the wheat family? If you answered no, you win! Buckwheat is not a member of the wheat family or any of the other cereal grasses. It is actually an herb that originated in central Asia and Siberia. It was introduced to Europe during the early fifteenth century, and the first settlers brought it to America.

How does it help? Buckwheat is gluten-free and loaded with health benefits, according to an extensive 2015 review article published in the *Journal of Agricultural and Food Chemistry*. It is a terrific source of fiber for weight control and digestive health. It also has hunger-taming protein without any of the cholesterol or saturated fat associated with animal protein. Plus, buckwheat contains eight essential amino acids, making it a complete protein source.

Other buckwheat benefits include fatigue-fighting iron, bone-building calcium, and immune-system-strengthening minerals such as manganese, magnesium, copper, and zinc. Buckwheat is also a good source of a flavonoid called rutin, which has been shown to protect against abnormal blood clots. Buckwheat is also high in omega-3 and omega-6 essential fatty acids.

How to use it? In the United States, buckwheat is usually milled into flour and used for pancakes. Unmilled buckwheat is known as buckwheat groats or kasha and has a pleasant, nutty flavor. Buckwheat flour can be made into a spaghetti-like noodle called soba, which can be served hot or cold.

Bulgur

What is it? I love bulgur because it cooks quickly. A staple of Middle Eastern cooking, bulgur is a form of whole wheat that has been parboiled, dried, ground into particles, and sifted into various sizes. None of its nutrition is lost in the process, however.

How does it help? Bulgur is high in fiber and packed with vitamins and minerals, especially energy-giving B vitamins and heart-healthy vitamin E.

How to use it? To add bulgur to a salad, simply rehydrate it in hot water and then drain it in a sieve. This is how the Middle Eastern side dish tabbouleh is prepared. It is then mixed with chopped parsley, onion, and tomato and bathed in a dressing of olive oil and fresh lemon juice. You also can use bulgur as a filler or serve it as a pilaf. Cooked bulgur makes a tasty hot cereal, especially when you add raisins and walnuts or almonds.

Use finely ground or medium bulgur in place of bread crumbs to give meatloaf more texture and fiber.

Farro

What is it? Chances are you've never heard of farro. Dating back to the ancient Roman Empire, farro is standard fare in many Mediterranean and Middle Eastern restaurants. It is a nutty-tasting grain and considered a gourmet specialty, but is available in most large supermarkets.

How does it help? Farro is lower in gluten than many other grains, and it's among the highest-fiber grains you can eat. Among its other virtues, it is brimming with B vitamins, zinc, iron, antioxidants, and even a good dose of protein.

How to use it? Farro makes a great side dish and can be used in any recipe that calls for grains.

Kamut

What is it? Kamut (pronounced ka-MOOT) is a large grain, called a "giant" wheat.

How does it help? One of the biggest benefits of kamut is that it's low-glycemic. Particularly important for diabetics, athletes, and dieters, low-glycemic foods "release" glucose into the body more slowly than high-glycemic foods. This not only helps balance blood sugars—which is critical for diabetics—but also takes away that "empty" feeling that makes us want to eat more.

How to use it? You can use cooked kamut in salads, or serve it like pasta with just about any sauce. Puffed kamut, when crushed, makes a great binder for meatloaf.

Millet

What is it? For centuries, millet has been a central ingredient in the diets of people living in countries such as India, Africa, and Japan. You can find this ancient grain in health food stores and well-stocked supermarkets.

How does it help? A gluten-free grain, millet contains nearly 15 percent protein, B vitamins, and lots of minerals (particularly heart-healthy magnesium and bone-strengthening phosphorus), and it is high in fiber.

How to use it? Millet is tasty as cereal, in salad, or in pilaf.

Oats

What are they? The oat is a species of cereal grain grown for its seed.

How do they help? I use oatmeal in my detox program, along with quinoa, to help people cleanse and lose weight. It increases satiety (fullness) and it is high in fiber that flushes out your digestive tract. Oats are higher in protein than corn, rice, or wheat and are rich in minerals including manganese, selenium, magnesium, zinc, and copper—all powerful immune boosters. Oats are also naturally gluten-free; however, they can become contaminated with wheat, barley, or rye during the growing and/or manufacturing process. It's important to get 100 percent gluten-free oats (noted on the bag) if you have celiac disease or a gluten sensitivity. If you're not comfortable eating oats, it's fine to replace them with quinoa flakes.

How to use it? Oats have so many uses. Bake them into cookies, bars, and breads; use them as fillers in veggie burgers or meatloaf; sprinkle them over fish or poultry to form a nice crusty topping; or simply enjoy them as a warm hearty breakfast cereal with nuts and fruits in the morning.

Quinoa

What is it? Quinoa is grown as a grain primarily for its edible seeds.

How does it help? Quinoa is one of my favorite "grains." It is gluten-free and contains all eight essential amino acids, making it a perfect protein for a plant-based diet. It is a great source of lysine, an amino acid that plays a valuable role in cellular repair. Plus, quinoa is rich in the antioxidant vitamin E to help cleanse your system and give you glowing skin, hair, and nails. Quinoa also has high levels of manganese, magnesium, phosphorus, folate, copper, iron, and zinc. These essential vitamins, nutrients, and minerals help reduce blood sugar levels, keep the body healthy and strong, and keep your digestion running smoothly. A detailed 2017 review of quinoa published in *Molecular Nutrition and Food Research* describes how the nutrients in this grain contribute to its potential health benefits, especially in lowering the risk of cancer, cardiovascular disease, diabetes, and obesity.

How to use it? Use it in salads, add it to soups, create veggie burgers with it, use it instead of oats for a morning breakfast bowl, or eat it with nutritional yeast flakes for a cheesy-tasting side dish.

Spelt

What is it? Spelt is a variety of wheat that has gotten more attention recently with the surge of interest in whole grains.

How does it help? Spelt is lower in gluten than wheat, making it easier to digest, and has more protein and a broad range of amino acids. Spelt is among the grains considered to have significant health benefits in the prevention of cardiovascular disease, diabetes, and cancer because of its high antioxidant and phytochemical content, according to a 2016 report in *Critical Reviews in Food Science and Nutrition*.

How to use it? Spelt may be cooked much as you would cook other whole grains. Spelt is also available in ground form as spelt flour, which can be substituted for whole-wheat flour or other whole-grain flours in recipes.

What is it? The world's tiniest grain, teff is about the size of a poppy seed, and ranges in color from white to reddish brown. Teff is so tiny that it can't be processed like most grains, so it's almost always eaten in its whole form, bran and germ intact, giving it a super-healthy advantage.

How does it help? There's a lot of calcium and magnesium packed into this teensy grain; both minerals are required for bone health and healthy blood pressure, among other benefits. Teff also dishes up 13 percent of your daily requirement for protein. It is a great grain for people who want to avoid gluten.

How to use it? Teff can be found in gluten-free recipes for pancakes, breads, crepes, or waffles and is showing up in products such as cereal, snacks, wraps, and more. You can also use it as a binding agent in veggie burgers.

Grain (1 cup, uncooked)	Cooking Liquid (usually water or stock)	Directions	Approximate Simmer Time	Approximate Yield (cups cooked)
Buckwheat Groats	2 cups	Bring the water to a boil in a pot. Add the groats to the boiling water and reduce the temperature so the groats simmer over low heat.	Cover the pot and cook for 12 to 15 minutes. Stir every five minutes.	Serve when the groats absorb all the water and have a slightly chewy, yet tender taste. Yields 2 cups.
Bulgur	2 ½ cups	Place the bulgur in a bowl. Boil the water in a pot. Pour it over the bulgur, and cover.	Allow it to stand for about 30 minutes.	Drain the bulgur in a strainer, transfer it to a bowl, and fluff it with a fork. Yields 2 cups.
*Farro	2 ½ cups	Pour the water into a pot and boil. Stir in the farro. Reduce heat to a simmer.	Exact cooking time can vary from 15 to 40 minutes, depending on the type of farro you use and the texture you prefer.	Drain the farro in a strainer, transfer it to a bowl, and fluff it with a fork. Yields 2 cups.
Kamut	3 cups	Combine kamut with water in a pot and bring to a boil. Reduce heat to low.	Cover and simmer for about an hour, until grains are tender.	Drain the kamut in a strainer, transfer it to a bowl, and fluff it with a fork. Yields 2 cups.
Millet	2 cups	Toast the millet grains in a dry pan or skillet. Stir consistently for approximately 4 minutes to keep them from burning. Stir the millet into water and bring to a boil at medium-high heat. Lower the heat to simmer.	Cover the pot to allow the millet to cook. Keep the lid on for at least 20 minutes. Remove the pan or pot of millet from the heat. Leave it covered and undisturbed for an additional 5 minutes.	Drain the millet in a strainer, transfer it to a bowl, and fluff it with a fork. Yields 2 cups.
Oats	2 cups	Bring the water to a boil; add the oats.	Cook about 5 minutes over medium heat; stir.	Yields 2 cups.

* It saves time to purchase semi-pearled and pearled farro, because these do not require soaking time. Other forms of farro must be soaked for 8 to 16 hours in the refrigerator.

(table continues)

Grain (1 cup, uncooked)	Cooking Liquid (usually water or stock)	Directions	Approximate Simmer Time	Approximate Yield (cups cooked)
Quinoa	2 cups	Add quinoa to water. Bring to a boil over high heat.	Reduce the heat to low, cover, and simmer for 15 minutes. Quinoa is done when it turns into ringlets. Remove the pot from the heat and let the quinoa sit, covered, for an additional 5 minutes.	After 5 minutes, remove the cover and use a fork to gently fluff the cooked quinoa. Yields 2 cups.
Rice, brown	2 ½ cups	Bring rice and water to a boil.	Reduce heat to low and simmer, covered, until the rice is tender and most of the liquid has been absorbed, about 40 to 50 minutes.	Let stand 5 minutes, then fluff with a fork. Yields 3 cups.
Spelt	3 ½ cups	Soak spelt berries in water for 1 hour, or even overnight is fine. Combine spelt berries and water in a pot and bring to a boil.	Reduce heat, cover, and simmer until tender, about 45 minutes.	Drain the spelt in a strainer, transfer it to a bowl, and fluff it with a fork. Yields 2 cups.
Teff	3 cups	Add the teff to a pot with the water and bring to a boil on high heat.	Once the teff is boiling, reduce the heat to low and cover the pot. Allow the teff to cook for 15 to 20 minutes.	Drain the teff in a strainer, transfer it to a bowl, and fluff it with a fork. Yields 2 cups.

When you combine super grains with other foods, such as vegetables and spices, you create fabulous super meals that allow you to eat in a way that is good for your body and keeps weight off. So let's stop being fearful of carbs once and for all, shall we? The super grains listed above will keep you full, add ample levels of protein and fiber to your diet, and make you forever change your view on carbohydrates.

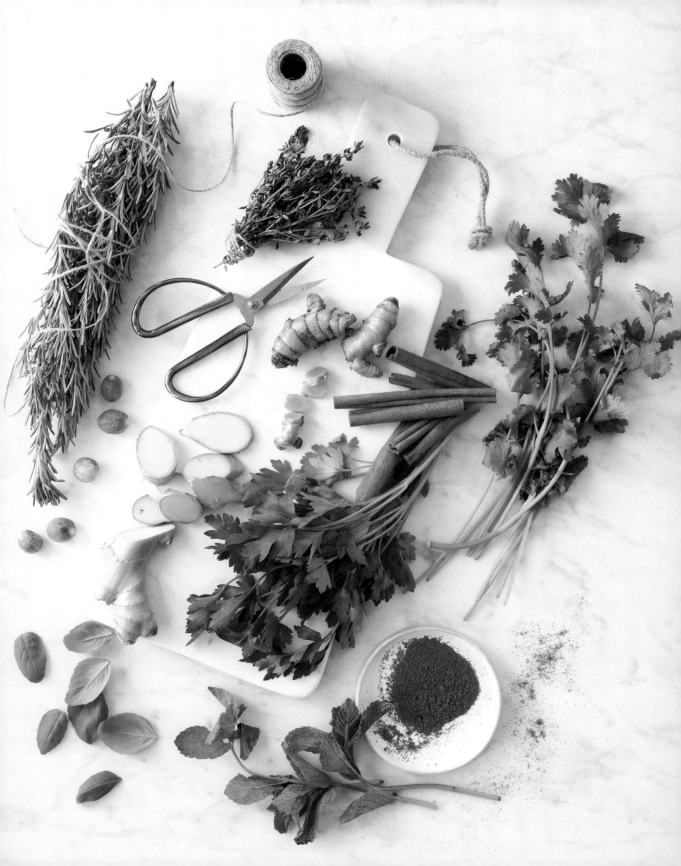

CHAPTER 9

Super Herbs and Spices

Over the years, and after many trips abroad, I've learned how to cook with herbs and spices, combining them in flavorful ways that reduce or even eliminate my need for salt. But these spices and herbs are more than just flavor boosters—they are super nutritional powerhouses. Think about it: spices and herbs come from plants, which means they are rich sources of plant phytonutrients. Many phytonutrients have detoxifying, antioxidant, anti-inflammatory, or even anti-cancer properties. You probably don't realize it, but your spice rack is actually a natural pharmacy in your kitchen. You'll be meal prepping with various spices and herbs, including the following.

Basil

What is it? Derived from the Greek word meaning "royal," basil is a leafy plant that lives up to its pedigree. You can buy the whole fresh leaves or the dried version. Basil is also easy to grow in your garden or on a sunny windowsill.

How does it help? Basil was among the culinary herbs evaluated in 2016 by *Critical Reviews in Food Science and Nutrition* for its anti-diabetic, anti-inflammatory, anti-hyperlipidemic (cholesterol-regulating), and anti-hypertensive properties. Basil contains a wealth of nutrients: hefty amounts of vitamin K, calcium, iron, vitamin A, and antioxidant oils. The leaves are also packed with beta-caryophyllene, an anti-inflammatory compound that may treat conditions such as arthritis and inflammatory bowel disease.

How to use it? Basil is a delicious and aromatic ingredient used frequently in Greek, Italian, and Thai cuisine. I love to use it in pesto, with fish or poultry, to add sparkle to salads, or as a garnish. I also add fresh leaves to a large water container for a beautiful fresh flavor.

Cayenne

What is it? Made from dried pods of chili peppers, cayenne is probably the most widely available ground chili, known for its spicy hotness.

How does it help? Cayenne has medicinal powers that are derived from a chemical called capsaicin, the ingredient that gives peppers their heat. Generally, the hotter the pepper, the more capsaicin it contains. There are a lot of health benefits associated with the use of cayenne, including the reduction of blood platelet stickiness, a condition that can lead to abnormal blood clotting. Cayenne is also considered a natural pain-fighter, due to its anti-inflammatory qualities.

How to use it? Cayenne is used in many different regional styles of cooking. I like to add it to Italian, Asian, and Mexican dishes, whenever I want a little heat in my meal. It goes well with everything from eggs to a variety of sauces to my morning lemon water with turmeric.

Cilantro

What is it? Also known as Chinese parsley or fresh coriander, cilantro is the leaves and stem of the coriander plant; the seeds are referred to as coriander. It is one of the most widely used herbs in the world.

How does it help? Like cardamom, turmeric, and ginger, cilantro can help fight cardiovascular disease, as highlighted in a 2017 article in *Current Pharmaceutical Design*.

How to use it? There are so many ways to use cilantro: in guacamole, in a fresh tomato salsa, in a savory ceviche, in coleslaw for fish tacos, as an accent for meats and pasta, or as a fresh garnish on any dish.

Cinnamon

What is it? Cinnamon comes from the inner bark of a tree that predominantly grows in India, China, and Sri Lanka, and is ground to a powder or formed into sticks.

How does it help? Cinnamon is known to be antibacterial. That is why it is used to fight bad breath and help with digestion. It is also helps prevent the common cold and soothe sore throats. Cinnamon helps control high blood sugar too.

How to use it? Add cinnamon to your breakfast oats, grains, or meat marinades. Sprinkle it on roasted vegetables or sautéed leafy greens. Mix it into black bean dishes. It has a sweet flavor, so it's a great replacement for sugar. Cinnamon is one of my favorite spices and I tend to go overboard when using it because it's just so darn good.

Ginger

What is it? Used in many different ethnic cuisines, ginger comes from the fleshy roots (called rhizomes) of a tropical plant.

How does it help? Ginger is a powerful antioxidant and is known to improve circulation, ease nausea, prevent bloating, fight colds, and lessen pain due to arthritis. Scientists in India found that ginger reduces the risk of atherosclerosis, an artery-clogging condition.

How to use it? To prepare ginger, scrape off the brown skin (extra points if you use a spoon), then chop, slice, or grate the flesh, or even crush it in a garlic press. Use it in smoothies, cakes, cookies, other baked goods, teas, and Asian-inspired dishes, as well as pureeing it into dressings.

Mint

What is it? Plants in the *Mentha* genus include twenty-five different species with varieties such as peppermint and spearmint.

How does it help? Several clinical trials have found that peppermint may treat digestive disorders by relaxing the smooth muscles surrounding the intestines. An active component in peppermint is rosmarinic acid, which can help relieve asthma suffering by reducing inflammation. Peppermint tea can ease indigestion and bloating.

How to use it? With its cooling flavor, mint is a refreshing addition to salads, smoothies, and hot and cold beverages. You can also bake it into brownies—think mint chocolate chip anything! My go-to for mint is adding a mint tea bag to my water bottle, no need for hot water. You instantly have delicious flavored water that will help you to stay hydrated.

Nutmeg

What is it? Nutmeg is actually a big seed, however in the United States, nutmeg is usually found already ground. But you can also buy it in the seed form and grind it yourself.

How does it help? Nutmeg is loaded with medicinal benefits. Herbalists and natural health practitioners believe it can help relieve pain, soothe indigestion, strengthen brainpower, detoxify the body, boost skin health, reduce insomnia, strengthen immunity, and improve blood circulation.

How to use it? Nutmeg is frequently the secret ingredient in cookies and other baked goods, as well as fettuccine alfredo or any cream sauce; it gives an extra zing to eggnog.

Rosemary

What is it? Rosemary is a woody herb in the same family as mint. It grows easily in gardens.

How does it help? Rosemary has a long, impressive resume of health benefits. It appears to help boost memory, improve mood, reduce inflammation, relieve pain, protect the immune system, stimulate circulation, detoxify the body, protect the body from bacterial infections, prevent premature aging, and heal skin conditions. That's a lot of health power packed into one little herb.

How to use it? Rosemary is wonderful in garlic mashed potatoes; with roasted vegetables; on meats, poultry, and chicken; in marinara sauce; and in various other recipes. Rosemary tea makes an excellent mouthwash and is a good antiseptic gargle.

Thyme

What is it? Thyme is an herb from the mint family that you probably already have in your spice rack.

How does it help? One of the best uses of thyme is in tea. It helps stop coughing and soothes a sore throat. It may also strengthen immunity because of its well-researched benefits as a germ fighter.

How to use it? Thyme is an excellent ingredient to use when preparing meat or poultry. It also unites flavors and brings harmony to soups, stews, roasts, and sauces as well as salads and vinaigrettes. It's especially good with fresh corn.

Turmeric

What is it? A member of the ginger family, this spice is well known as a bitter, pungent, bright yellow flavoring found in curry dishes famous in the cuisines of India and other parts of Asia.

How does it help? One of the most widely studied spices, turmeric is an effective anti-inflammatory agent. It fights coughs, colds, asthma, and other bronchial-related illnesses. In Asian countries, it is popular as a remedy for liver disease. Turmeric contains curcumin, a natural anti-inflammatory chemical that is believed to help prevent Alzheimer's disease. Alzheimer's is linked to the formation of knots in the brain, known as "amyloid plaques," and research has shown that curcumin can cut down the formation of these knots.

How to use it? I like to incorporate turmeric in my everyday diet. The taste can be pretty strong, but it's great when combined with all of the following ingredients in this section. For example, turmeric, basil, and cayenne are spicy partners in many Indian dishes, and turmeric and ginger combine to make a delicious, healing tea. When you add turmeric to dishes, use black pepper too, because a compound in black pepper helps your body absorb turmeric's beneficial compounds.

Even alone, turmeric is delightful in soups, stews, and curries.

If you're not yet familiar with some of these spices, don't worry. Just have some of them on hand before you begin the plan, and follow the recipes. As I mentioned before, if this seems like a lot to buy all at once, I would say choose one or two, and then add in a couple at a time. Keep experimenting.

My goal is never to overwhelm you with the amount of ingredients. I truly want you to learn how to prep and cook with various herbs and spices. I know you will fall in love with how they flavor your food and make you feel. You won't even know you're on a weight-loss plan.

CHAPTER 10
Super Beverages

You've heard the phrase "You are what you eat," but guess what? You are also what you drink. Your beverage choices play a major role in your health—and your weight.

When investigators from the University of North Carolina School of Public Health scrutinized dietary trends around the world, they discovered a surge in the consumption of sugar-laden foods—particularly beverages and particularly in the United States. Over the last ten years, the number of calories the average American takes in from soft drinks and fruit drinks has jumped from 70 calories a day to 136. And those calories add up: an extra 66 calories per day translates to more than six pounds per year. Studying food trends around the world, investigators from the University of North Carolina School of Public Health found a surge in consumption of sugar-laden foods—particularly beverages, especially in the United States.

What you drink can make or break your diet. And no wonder—the average 12-ounce can of regular soda contains the equivalent of 8 to 9 teaspoons of granulated sugar.

Here's the lowdown on what to drink, and not to drink, while following my 28-day plan.

Refresh and Hydrate: Detox Waters

I'm relentless when it comes to telling people to drink more water. The recommended amount of water to drink daily is 8 to 10 cups, and the question I seem to get most often in relation to water is *how* to go about drinking that much.

The primary complaints I hear about drinking enough water are: it's boring, water bottles run out and then don't get refilled, and water tastes bad.

If any of these complaints sound familiar, know that you are not alone. Even I struggle with drinking enough water, especially when I'm super busy. That is why I created my detox waters, which makes water easier to drink.

So how do you make detox water? Simple! Just buy a few mason jars, slice up whatever fruits you have around the house, or herbs such as basil and rosemary, and fill your jars with fruit and water. You will drink more water with detox waters because they are pretty to look at, taste delicious, and can be refilled two to three times without changing the fruit in them. They are best when allowed to sit overnight in the fridge. Simply prep all your waters the night before and have them ready to take to work the next day.

You'll notice that these waters are a conversation starter. I like to bring my large mason jar with fruit or lemon and mint around with me when I'm out, just to see how many people come up and start talking to me. Hey, that's even how I got talking to some celebrities! You'll be amazed at how many people want to know what you're drinking, simply because of how many people also struggle to drink enough water.

Finally, detox waters provide you with the vitamins and minerals found in fruit without the calories of eating fruit. Don't get me wrong, fruit is an excellent snack and should be incorporated into your diet once or twice a day, but sometimes we want the nutrients from fruit when we're already full or when we're watching how much we eat. The fruit leaches out its nutritional goodness into the water, and you get to drink in all its amazing health benefits. One more point: If you're a soda drinker (even diet sodas), please get off them now, as they are as bad as—if not worse than—normal sodas. Drinking my detox waters will help you do so.

Here are my favorite detox waters:

Citrus Spa Water

Ingredients
4 strawberries, sliced
1 lemon, sliced
½ cucumber, sliced
Handful of fresh mint

Directions

1. Place all the ingredients in a large mason jar and fill with cold, filtered water.

2. Allow it to sit overnight in your refrigerator to let the ingredients infuse into the water.

Rosemary Lime Water

Ingredients
2 limes, sliced
Handful of fresh rosemary sprigs

Directions

1. Place all the ingredients in a large mason jar and fill with cold, filtered water.

2. Allow it to sit overnight in your refrigerator to let the ingredients infuse into the water.

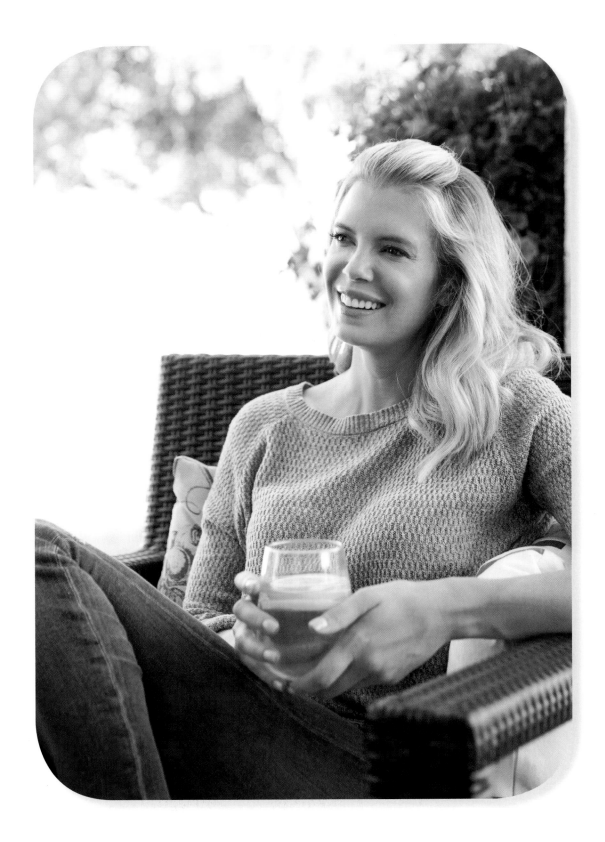

Ginger-Licious Water

Ingredients

1-inch piece ginger, peeled and cut into thin slices
Handful of fresh blueberries

Directions

1. Place all the ingredients in a large mason jar and fill with cold, filtered water. My go-to tip for peeling the ginger is to use a spoon against the skin. Begin peeling it as you would with a peeler and you'll find that the tip of the spoon reaches the hard-to-reach spots a peeler can't.
2. Allow it to sit overnight in your refrigerator to let the ingredients infuse into the water.

Strawberry Zinger Water

Ingredients

4 strawberries, sliced
2 limes, sliced

Directions

1. Place all the ingredients in a large mason jar and fill with cold, filtered water.
2. Allow it to sit overnight in your refrigerator to let the ingredients infuse into the water.

Pomegranate Water

Ingredients

1 tablespoon fresh blueberries
1 tablespoon pomegranate seeds
Handful of fresh basil leaves

Directions

1. Place all the ingredients in a large mason jar and fill with cold, filtered water.

2. Allow it to sit overnight in your refrigerator to let the ingredients infuse into the water.

Orange Berry Water

Ingredients
1 orange, washed and sliced
1 tablespoon fresh raspberries, washed

Directions
1. Place all the ingredients in a large mason jar and fill with cold, filtered water.
2. Allow it to sit overnight in your refrigerator to let the ingredients infuse into the water.

Brew Up Health: Herbal Teas

Another excellent way to hydrate your body is to drink herbal teas. They have therapeutic effects that can enhance health, treat minor ailments, reduce our toxic burden (caused by pollution, chemicals in food, alcohol, and secondhand smoke), and can even help prevent disease. This is because herbs have long had medicinal value and were humankind's first "drugs."

Technically, an herbal tea is a water-based infusion of the flower, leaves, or other soft parts of an herb. Herbal teas are a cinch to prepare—simply pour hot water over the herbs, or tea bags, and let them steep a few minutes until they are ready to drink. You remove the herbs or tea bag and, as you take a sip, you receive gentle healing for whatever ails you. You can enjoy an herbal tea by itself, or mix several in a blend. In addition to the health benefits of the following herbs, the simple act of drinking tea can be a calming ritual.

So many herbal teas have proven medicinal value. Here are a few of my favorites:

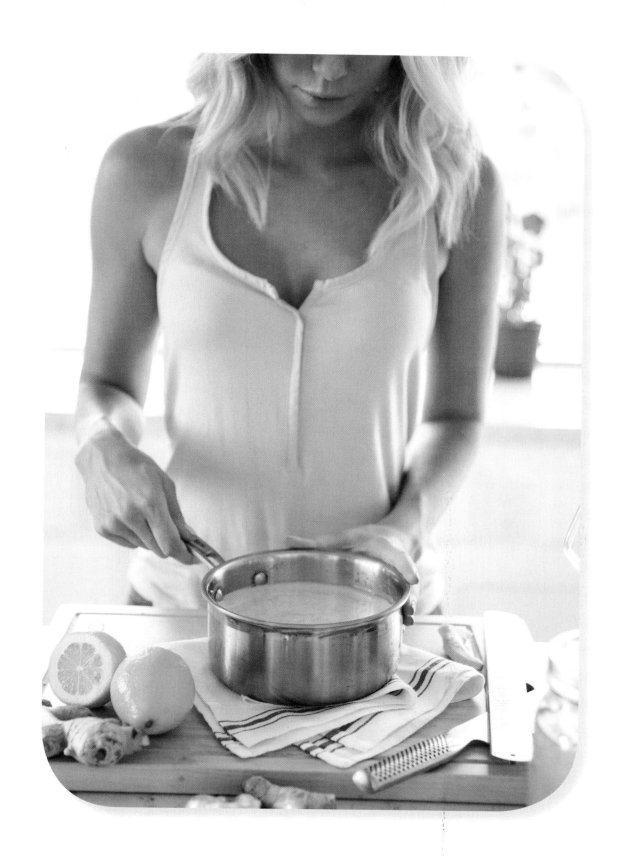

Fennel tea. Fennel tea is great for improving digestion and relieving constipation because it works on the internal muscles that help food move through your system. It is also a diuretic that helps your kidneys flush out toxins. It's best to drink fennel tea after meals to prevent post-meal bloating.

There's more good news: Fennel tea can act as an appetite suppressant, according to a Korean study published in 2015 in the journal *Clinical Nutrition Research*. Nine overweight women were given either fennel tea or, as a placebo, fenugreek tea (another type of herbal tea). After drinking a given tea, a lunch buffet was served, and the researchers analyzed the women's food consumption, appetite, hunger, fullness, and desire to eat. Both the fennel tea and fenugreek tea decreased hunger, led to less food consumption, and increased feelings of fullness compared to the placebo tea. The researchers concluded that both herbal teas worked significantly and effectively to curb appetite among overweight women.

Peppermint tea. Peppermint is a valuable herb that has many uses, including relieving intestinal upset, traveler's diarrhea, anxiety, and tension. Like fennel tea, it is great to drink after a heavy meal because it will help you de-bloat.

Scientists from the U.S. Department of Agriculture found that peppermint has significant antimicrobial and antiviral activities, strong antioxidant and antitumor actions, and antiallergenic potential.

Dandelion tea. Although I usually stay on the slim side, I often have a bloated tummy, which doesn't make me look or feel great. As a remedy, I reach for dandelion tea. Its leaves acts as a powerful diuretic, helping the body clear toxins through the kidneys. The root stimulates the liver to clear toxins by releasing bile into the digestive tract.

Ginger tea. This delicious tea is commonly used to alleviate motion sickness, nausea, and indigestion. It can also relieve headaches, as it is believed to relax blood vessels in the head and activate the body's natural pain relievers. In addition, ginger can reduce prostaglandins—hormones that cause inflammation in the body.

Green tea. This popular tea contains polyphenols—natural chemicals thought to lower cholesterol, act as antioxidants, protect against cancer, and help your body burn fat. A 2017 study in *Phytomedicine* reported that green tea also has antibacterial properties.

Here are my favorite recipes for homemade herbal teas.

Goji Berry Tea

Ingredients
1 tablespoon dried goji berries
1 quart water

Directions
1. Place the goji berries and water into a pot and bring to a boil. Turn off heat and allow the mixture to brew for 10 to 20 minutes. Serve warm or cold.
2. Store in your refrigerator, with goji berries still in the water, once it has come to room temperature.

Immune-Boosting Tea

Ingredients
1 quart water
1-inch piece ginger, peeled and thinly sliced
½ tablespoon turmeric powder, or 1 tablespoon thinly sliced fresh turmeric root
Juice of 1 lemon
1 tablespoon honey
¼ teaspoon black pepper

Directions
1. Place all ingredients into a pot and bring to a boil. Turn off heat and allow to brew with lid on for 20 minutes. Serve warm or cold.
2. Store in your refrigerator once it has come to room temperature.

Turmeric Tea

Ingredients
3 cups homemade almond milk (see p. 119)
1 tablespoon coconut oil (optional)
1 teaspoon turmeric powder
1 teaspoon ground cinnamon
1 teaspoon grated ginger
¼ teaspoon vanilla extract
Pinch of black pepper

Directions
1. Place all ingredients in a small pot and bring to a gentle boil, stirring to combine. Reduce heat to low and simmer for around 10 minutes. The longer you let it steep, the more intense the flavors will be.
2. Use a nut milk bag to strain if there are large pieces of the grated ginger.

Note: This quick, simple drink can help you sleep at night, will give you energy the next morning, and can be used as a coffee replacement. You can serve it hot or chilled over ice. I'll even add a shot of espresso to this in the morning if I really need a pick-me-up. It tastes great after dinner too, if you're craving something sweet or need a healthy after-dinner drink.

Sleepy Time Tea

Ingredients
1 quart water
20 fresh lemon balm leaves or 2 tablespoons dried lemon balm

Directions
1. Place the water and lemon balm in a pot and bring to a boil.
2. Turn the heat off and let the mixture steep at least thirty minutes, or overnight.

Note: Lemon balm is an incredible herb that has a wide range of uses, including reducing stress, anxiety, and indigestion. It can also improve your sleep, especially when brewed with the herbs chamomile and/or valerian.

Non-Dairy Milks

You may have heard that dairy milk is out, soy milk is out, and nut milk is in. I want to take a moment to explain why this is and why certain store-bought nut milks aren't always your best choice either.

When I was growing up in Boulder, Colorado, every Wednesday morning the milkman would come and deliver fresh milk in glass bottles, straight from the farm. We ordered around four bottles, which would last us until the next week. We'd place the empty bottles into a little mailbox-type place that the milkman could access from the outside of our house and we could access from the inside. This milk was luscious—creamy and great-tasting.

Eventually the milkman stopped coming. I don't remember the details, but it was either because the milk delivery got too expensive or he went out of business. But this was also the time that pasteurized milk became popular—and cheap. Without our weekly milk deliveries, we bought 1 percent or skim milk (since low-fat foods were all the rage then) from the grocery store in plastic gallon containers. Why am I sharing this story with you? Because this is the way our world has changed, especially when it comes to food. Milk that was natural and delivered straight from the farm was not nearly as unhealthy as mass-produced milk. Cows are pumped up with hormones and antibiotics and they're fed unnatural diets designed purely to make them produce more milk. Nowadays, milk is overloaded with lactose (the sugar in milk) because of the modern ways in which cattle are raised. The human body has a very hard time digesting this much lactose. Acne, bloating, fatigue, and other conditions are all common side effects of eating processed dairy foods. After I started drinking mass-produced milk, I suffered from absolutely terrible acne, and I went on Accutane three times. It wasn't until I cut out dairy that my skin finally cleared up.

I'm not here to give you a lecture about milk and dairy, however. Instead, I just want you to know that commercially produced almond milk and soy milk are not necessarily that much better. I'm going to ruffle a lot of feathers by saying that, but stay with me!

When I began my health journey, I switched from cow's milk to soy milk. I put it in coffee, tea, and smoothies. I had it with cereal, and I drank glasses of it. Then I learned that soy milk isn't really that great for you either. It has been blamed for fatigue, stomach disorders, weight gain, and hormone problems. Plus, many people are allergic to soy. No wonder food manufacturers started labeling their products "soy-free."

Alarmed, I switched to almond milk and other nut milks. What's so bad about almond milk, then? It's made from almonds and water . . . right?

Well, yes and no. Almond milk lasts for weeks in your fridge, as well as on the shelves, without spoiling. If you've ever made your own nut milk, though, you know that it lasts only a few days before going bad. Commercially produced almond milk has something in it to preserve it, for sure. No biggie, right? After all, almonds are good for you. They're an incredibly good source of healthy fats, vitamin E, and protein, and they make a great healthy snack. The problem is, these milks typically have only about one small handful of almonds in them per carton! So where is the rest of the milk coming from and why is it so thick and creamy?

Commercial almond milk is a mixture of almonds, water, sugar, flavorings, and carrageenan (a thickener). Often the milk contains added vitamins, which are not necessarily good for you, since it's better to get your vitamins from food, not from a product that says "fortified with B vitamins." Essentially, you're paying a high price for a watered-down milk with extra nasties that don't digest well in your body.

I don't want to scare you off all milk, but I'd like you to read labels and see what goes into commercially produced rice milk, hemp milk, almond milk, and cow's milk. You might be a bit shocked at how many additives are in them. One is carrageenan, a gelatin-like substance extracted from red seaweed, which may cause mild to severe asthma attacks, rashes, and digestive discomfort. Some companies can be tricky and add in things like sugar in different names (usually ending in "-ose"), as well as canola oil.

Here are some examples of ingredients in popular non-dairy milks:

- Silk Almond Milk: almond milk (filtered water, almonds), cane sugar, salt, natural flavor, locust bean gum, sunflower lecithin, gellan gum, calcium carbonate, vitamin E acetate, zinc gluconate, vitamin A palmitate, riboflavin (B$_2$), vitamin B$_{12}$, vitamin D$_2$

- Blue Diamond Almond Breeze: almond milk (filtered water, almonds), evaporated cane juice, calcium carbonate, potassium citrate, salt, sunflower lecithin, gellan gum, vitamin A palmitate, vitamin D$_2$, D-alpha-tocopherol (natural vitamin E)
- Trader Joe's Almond Milk: almond milk (filtered water, almonds), tricalcium phosphate, salt, gellan gum, dipotassium phosphate, xanthan gum, natural flavors, sunflower lecithin, vitamin A palmitate, vitamin D$_2$, dl-alpha tocopherol acetate (vitamin E)

To me, those are a lot of ingredients in what should be almonds and water! Remember, I'm not telling you to avoid these products; I'm advising you to be savvy. Look for the following labels: organic, non-GMO, and unsweetened. And choose products made with gellan gum over carrageenan (for the thickener). Of course, the best alternative is to ...

Make Your Own Nut Milk

Making your own nut milk is so simple and tastes better than anything else! The key is to soak your nuts or seeds overnight, then rinse and drain them before mixing them with the filtered water. *Don't forget this step.*

Add the rinsed and drained nuts with your water in a high-speed blender, mixing for 1 to 2 minutes or until the mixture is thick and creamy. Then use a nut milk bag, cheese cloth, or thin dish towel over a container to strain the milk out. To make it taste even more delicious, add 1 to 2 pitted Medjool dates, a pinch of salt, and a dash of organic vanilla extract. Or add a teaspoon of coconut oil, a pinch of Himalayan sea salt, and a date, and you have a very decadent and rich-tasting milk. Love chocolate milk? Add 1 to 2 tablespoons raw cacao powder.

Store homemade milk in an airtight container in your fridge. It will last up to 5 days. Use organic ingredients when possible.

Here are several ways to make your own nut, grain, or seed milk:

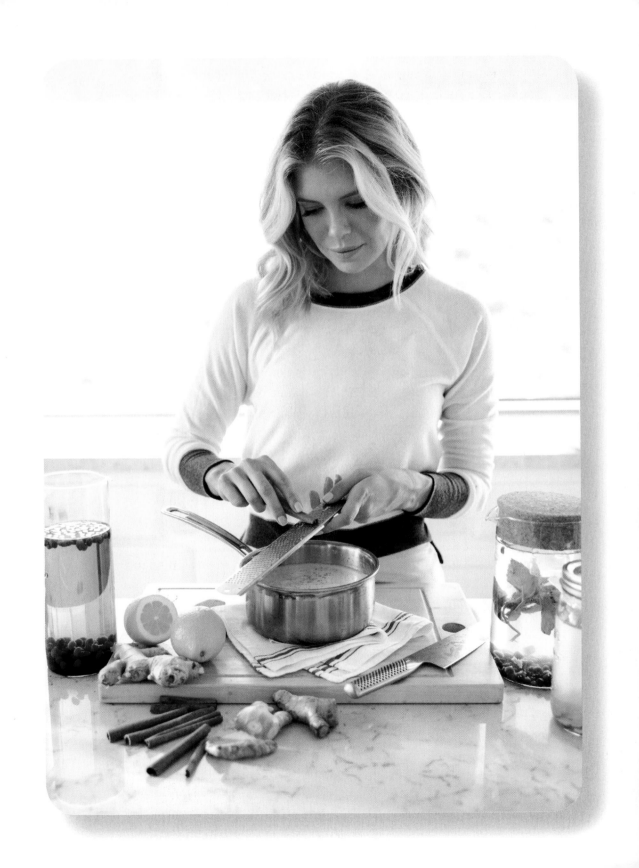

Almond Milk: 1 cup almonds, 3 cups water. Blend 1 to 2 minutes on highest speed. Strain.

Sunflower Seed Milk: 1 cup sunflower seeds, 3 to 4 cups water. Blend 1 minute on highest speed. Strain.

Rice Milk: 1 cup brown rice, 3 cups water. Blend 1 to 2 minutes. Strain.

Hemp Seed Milk: 1 cup shelled hemp seeds, 3 cups water. No need to pre-soak the hemp seeds. Blend 1 to 2 minutes on highest speed. Strain.

Brazil Nut Milk: 1 cup Brazil nuts, 3 cups water. Blend 2 minutes. Strain.

Cashew Nut Milk: 1 cup raw cashews, 3 cups water. Blend 1 to 2 minutes. Strain.

How easy is all this? Enjoy these milks like they're the best beverages you've ever tasted. Cook with them too, and use them as a base for smoothies. The possibilities are endless.

The Not-So-Good Beverages

Coffee

You've probably heard that coffee isn't good for you. It's acidic, it can be toxic, it prevents you from absorbing nutrients, and it can be a caloric bomb if you add milk and sugar, or slurp on those special coffee concoctions at your favorite coffeehouse. And you've also probably heard that coffee is good to drink daily because it has high levels of antioxidants, helps promote bowel movements, can help you burn fat, and more.

So, to coffee or not to coffee? That is the question. I get asked this question every day. Here is the simple truth: I can't tell you if you should be having coffee or not. It really is a personal choice. If you want to have it during the four-week plan, do so. Or if you can, skip it. It's important to note, though, if you are having more than one cup a day or must have it served with milk, and especially sugar, then it's best to cut down as much as possible, if not altogether. Needing multiple cups of coffee tends to mean that you are nutrient-deficient and not getting enough quality sleep, which coffee will never solve. If you drink it with milk and/or sugar, then your body is not necessarily craving the caffeine but more likely the sugar, which is highly addictive and bad for the body.

Ideally, skipping coffee is best during the 28 days. The wonderful super meals on this plan will nourish your body with antioxidants, provide you with energy, and keep you satisfied. That being said, if you want to have one cup of coffee a day while on the plan, then I am going to give you the go-ahead. Here are a few suggestions to follow:

- Drink only one cup a day.
- Use only non-dairy milk to flavor your coffee, and in small doses. Lattes and cappuccinos are not recommended.
- Do not use coffee to replace any meals or keep yourself full.
- Use a *very* small bit of stevia to sweeten your coffee if you absolutely must—no sugar or honey (but ideally no sweetener because it can heighten your craving for sweets). Alternatively, cinnamon is a wonderful additive instead of sugar.
- For an energy boost, add super ingredients, such as maca powder, baobab, and cinnamon to your foods, rather than depend on coffee and the caffeine it contains.
- If you feel you need a second cup of coffee during the day, try a cup of green tea, and make sure you've had enough water, as cravings for caffeine can mean you're dehydrated.

I don't believe in setting incredibly strict rules because it automatically makes our mind want whatever it is we are not permitting ourselves. If you love coffee, then keep having it, but try to wean yourself off it slowly so that you are having a maximum of one cup a day. If you're going to drink coffee on this plan, make sure to drink lots of water and herbal teas the rest of the day. I would suggest swapping out extra cups of coffee for caffeinated teas, such as black or green. Eventually you might find that you don't even really crave coffee anymore. I love my one cup of coffee a day and have it either with breakfast or a little bit after. I always make it with a dash of almond milk and mix it with the super ingredients listed previously. These strategies have weaned me off the need to drink multiple cups of coffee each day and have helped many of my clients, including those who would drink up to six cups a day! So please listen to your body here. At the same time, challenge yourself to not drink it. Coffee is an incredibly addicting substance, but I know you can absolutely stop drinking it if you put your mind to it.

Alcohol

Now let's switch topics and talk about alcohol. Over the next four weeks, there will be times when you're invited out for dinner, drinks, and parties. Or you might just have a hard day and want to relax with a glass of wine or beer at home. I get it. Life can be stressful, and we like to relax with alcohol. At the same time, life can be fun, and we celebrate with alcohol.

However, drinking alcohol could lead to "pound a month" weight gain, says a British study. The study found that the typical Brit guzzles more than 1,000 calories a week in alcohol alone, meaning a couch potato might pack on a pound of weight every three and a half weeks. The average Brit goes through more than two liters of alcohol a week—that's the equivalent of about 8.5 large glasses of wine.

Another study, published in 2016 by Spanish researchers in the journal *Nutrients,* showed that if people replaced one beer with one serving of water a day, they'd be less likely to become obese, and in fact could lose weight over a four-year period. (Maybe that's what the Brits should do! I'm half British, after all, so this advice is good for me too.)

There are several reasons alcoholic beverages cause weight gain. One is that alcohol loosens your inhibitions, making it more likely that you'll eat and drink more. Add on the hangover and wanting that greasy breakfast, a caloric bomb, to make you feel better. Another has to do with metabolism. When you drink alcohol, your liver goes to work metabolizing those cocktails and stops its regular job of burning fat. Finally, alcoholic beverages are high in sugar, which is high in calories and turned into fat quite easily.

If you're following my 28-day plan and want to really see results, then cutting out alcohol is key. Whether you want to lose weight, increase energy, sleep better, save money, or be more productive, cutting out the booze for four weeks will help you meet your goals faster.

Having said that, if you absolutely can't give it up, here's what I recommend:

- Choose one night a week when you'll enjoy alcohol, but stick with two drinks only.
- Skip alcoholic drinks that contain sugary ingredients, such as cranberry juice, sugary soft drinks, mixers, and tonic, and instead go with red or white wine, vodka soda, or tequila with soda and lime.
- Alternate your drinks with water, so that you slow down your drinking, prevent dehydration, and resist the temptation to have more than two drinks over the course of the evening.

Your results will not be as great if you don't skip the alcohol. However, if you're looking to make an overall lifestyle change, this is a good way to follow the plan.

Remember: You are what you drink, so lead with water and choose your other beverages wisely.

Part Three

The 28-Day Meal Prep Weight-Loss Diet

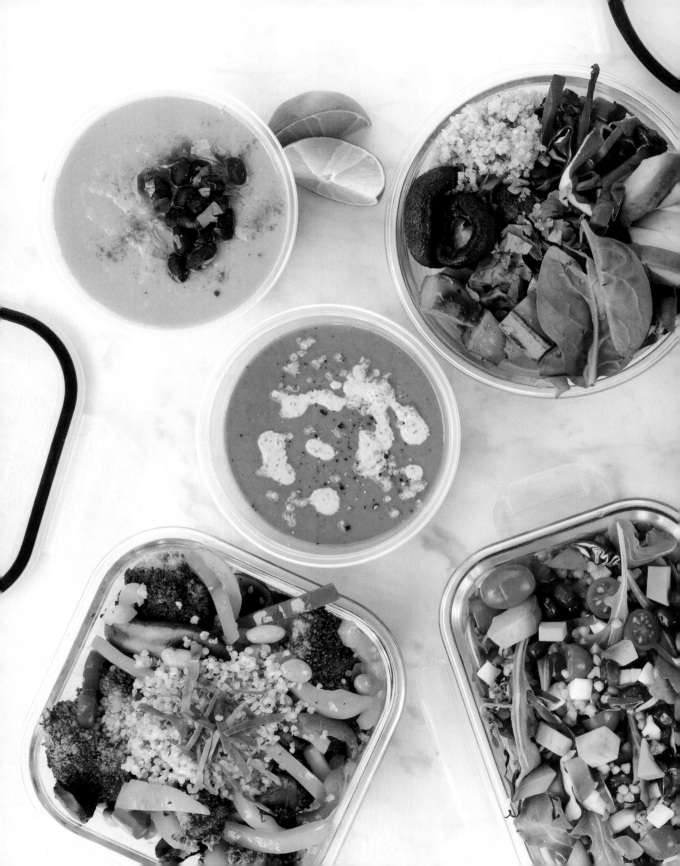

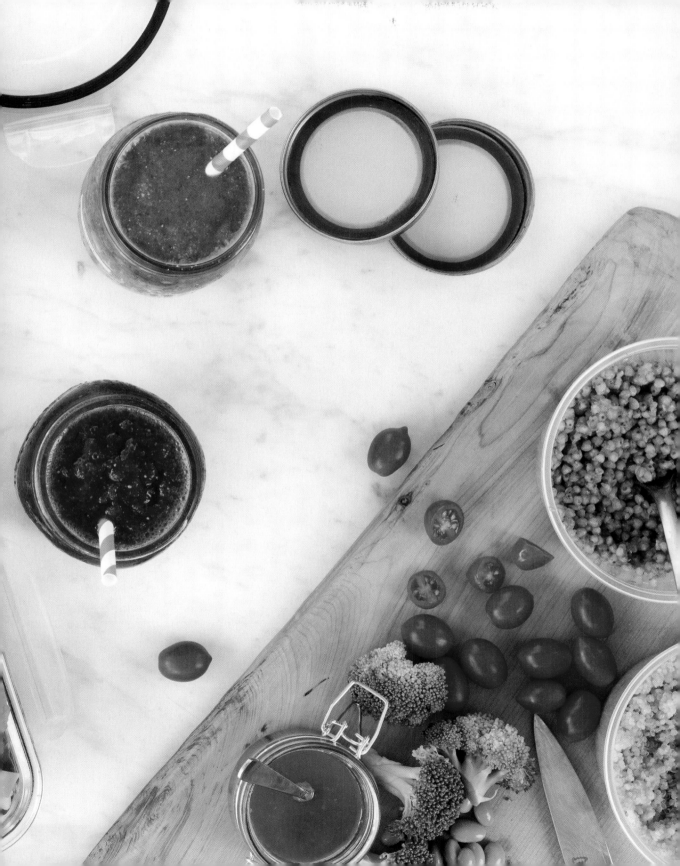

CHAPTER 11

Week One—Souping and Smoothies

Now we start the plan. Each week, I give you:

- A week's worth of menus—breakfast, lunch, dinner, and snacks. These menus outline what to eat each day, Monday through Sunday. Most of the meals are designed to be used as leftovers—a crucial, time-saving component of meal prepping.
- A shopping list for the week.
- A week's worth of recipes.
- Prep instructions for your prep day—which will typically be Sunday. Often, the prep instructions will mirror and repeat the recipe instructions. I provide both in case you want to fix some of the recipes on other days instead of on your prep day. (Some people

like to cook most days of the week. I understand that, because cooking can be relaxing and provide fresher food.)

Week one focuses on souping and smoothies. This will give your digestive system a rest, pump your body with lots of high-nutrition liquids, and kick-start your weight loss. It's also a great way to ease into meal prepping, as there isn't as much to do, so you'll get the hang of it quickly. Nothing like overwhelming you off the bat to make you want to quit! Nope, this plan eases you into things so that you'll truly enjoy the routine of prepping your food each Sunday and the benefits you'll get from doing so.

One thing to keep in mind: if you feel the recipes require an overwhelming amount of prep, then I suggest keeping your snack prep to a minimum. The snack recipes I've provided are all nutritious and very tasty; however, I know how it feels when you don't want to do any more cooking than absolutely necessary. If that's the case, stick with a handful of raw nuts and a piece of fruit, hummus and carrot sticks, or extra portions of any of the meals you are creating for breakfast, lunch, or dinner. Doing so will cut down on your prep time.

Please note that the recipes have been written so that you can make multiple meals at once, instead of cooking each and every day. The quantities might seem a bit high when you look at them; however, you'll make them all in one sitting, then portion them out in containers for the week. This saves a lot of time and helps you to grab-and-go with meal prepped food, instead of buying something naughty.

Let's get to it!

WEEK ONE MEAL PLAN

	Monday	Tuesday	Wednesday	Thursday	Friday	Saturday	Sunday
Breakfast	Super Meal Smoothie	Super Meal Smoothie	Super Meal Smoothie	Ginger Beet Smoothie	Ginger Beet Smoothie	Ginger Beet Smoothie	Ginger Beet Smoothie or Super Meal Smoothie
Lunch	Pomegranate, Arugula Salad	Pomegranate, Arugula Salad	Pomegranate, Arugula Salad	Buddha Bowl	Buddha Bowl	Buddha Bowl	Buddha Bowl
Dinner	Nikki's Thai Sweet Potato Soup	Nikki's Thai Sweet Potato Soup	Nikki's Thai Sweet Potato Soup	Broccoli Soup with Quinoa and Cilantro Sauce	Broccoli Soup with Quinoa and Cilantro Sauce	Broccoli Soup with Quinoa and Cilantro Sauce	Sensational Stir-Fry

Snacks: Choose 1–2 per day from pages 237–249

Grocery List for Week One

Staples, Spices, and Super Ingredients

This list of staples, spices, and super ingredients might look intense to buy at one time, but note that these are items to have on hand for the entire four weeks. Remember, you don't need to get everything all at once. Pick out a few spices and super ingredients you'd like to try in week one, then add more once you get used to cooking with each ingredient.

Spices

Black pepper

Cayenne

Cinnamon

Cumin

Paprika

Red pepper flakes

Salt

Turmeric powder

Vanilla extract

Xanthan gum, 1 small package

Super Ingredients

Baobab, 6-ounce package

Bee pollen, 6-ounce package

Cacao nibs, 8-ounce bag

Chia seeds, 12-ounce package

Flaxseed, ground, 6-ounce package

Goji berries, 6-ounce package

Hemp seeds, 6-ounce package

Maca powder, 6-ounce package

Pumpkin seeds, 1 2-ounce package

Raw cacao powder, 16-ounce package

Spirulina, 6-ounce package

Wheatgrass powder, 4.2-ounce container

Other Staples

Agave syrup, honey, or maple syrup (small bottles, usually around 12 ounces)

Apple cider vinegar, 16-ounce bottle

Baking soda

129

Balsamic vinegar, 16-ounce
bottle

Coconut oil, 16-ounce bottle

Coconut sugar, 16-ounce
package

Liquid aminos (such as Bragg's)

Nutritional yeast flakes, 5-ounce
jar

Olive oil, 16-ounce bottle

Reduced-sodium soy sauce,
15-ounce bottle

Stevia, 16-ounce package

Tahini, 16-ounce jar

Unsweetened coconut flakes,
7-ounce package

White miso

White wine vinegar

Items for This Week

Vegetables

Arugula, 16-ounce package

Avocado, 2

Basil, 1 small package

Beet, 1

Bell pepper, 1 (any color)

Broccoli, 2 small heads or
1 large, plus 1 small bag of
broccoli florets

Carrot, 1

Cauliflower, 1 head

Celery, 1 bunch

Cherry tomatoes, 1 small
package

Cilantro, 1 bunch

Cremini mushrooms, 2 pounds

Cucumbers, 2

Frozen shelled edamame,
14-ounce package

Fennel, 1 bulb

Garlic, 1 bulb

Ginger, 2 to 3 fresh roots

Kale, 16-ounce package

Leek, 1

Onions, 2

Parsley, 1 bunch

Portobello mushroom, 1

Red cabbage, 1 small head

Spinach, 1 to 2 16-ounce
packages

Sweet potatoes, 2 medium

Fruits

Bananas, 2

Lemon, 1

Limes, 3

Pineapple, 4 cartons of fresh
chunks or 1 package of frozen
(unsweetened)

Pomegranate seeds, 2 fruits or
1 cup of prepackaged seeds

Strawberries, 1 pint

Fresh fruits to have on hand for
snacking

Grains

Buckwheat groats, 16-ounce
package

Quinoa, 16-ounce package

Additional

Coconut milk, full fat,
2 13.5-ounce cans

Coconut water, 34 fluid ounces

Vegetable stock, 32 fluid ounces

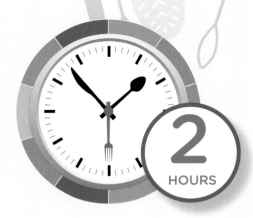

Overview:
Meal Prep Timing—Week One

5 minutes: Prepare area

5 minutes: Prepare quinoa for cooking

15–20 minutes: Prep smoothies

30 minutes: Prep salads

30 minutes: Prep soups

15 minutes: Prep Sensational Stir-Fry

10 minutes: Clean up

< 2 hours: total time*

* With optional snacks: Add 10 to 20 minutes to the total time.

Meal Prep for Week One

1. Prep your grains for the week. Follow package directions or see instructions on pages 95–96.

2. Prep your smoothies. Have a supply of large, freezable baggies ready. The prep instructions below will give you six smoothies total, as you get to choose which smoothie you'd like for your last day.

   - For the Super Meal Smoothie: You'll be prepping and freezing three smoothies for the week.

     - Review the recipe.

     - Divide ingredients equally among three baggies.

     - Seal each baggie and freeze.

     - When you're ready for your smoothie, place the frozen ingredients in your blender, add the coconut water, coconut oil, and ice, and blend well.

   - For the Ginger Beet Smoothie: You'll be prepping and freezing three smoothies for the week.

     - Review the recipe.

     - Portion out three servings and place each serving in a baggie.

     - Seal each baggie and freeze.

     - When you're ready for your smoothie, place the frozen ingredients in your blender, add the coconut oil, water, and ice, and blend well.

3. Prep your salads.

   - For the Pomegranate-Arugula Salad: You'll be prepping and refrigerating three servings.

     - Review the recipe.

- Chop your vegetables and divide your ingredients equally among three containers and seal.

- Portion your salad dressing into three small containers (about 2 tablespoons each).

- When you are ready to serve this salad, add the avocado (or toasted pumpkin seeds) and salad dressing.

- For the Buddha Bowl: You'll be prepping and refrigerating four servings.

  - Review the recipe.

  - Roast the sweet potatoes and mushrooms according to recipe instructions.

  - Arrange the spinach, mushrooms, sweet potatoes, ¼ cup of cooked quinoa, and cabbage in each bowl. Seal well and refrigerate.

  - When ready to serve, add avocado, drizzle with dressing, and top with chopped basil.

KEEPING YOUR AVOCADO FRESH

Like apples, avocados start to brown once you cut them, which can be a pain when you are trying to meal prep. The best way to keep avocados fresh and green is to cut them right before eating your meal. If this is not possible, squeeze fresh lemon juice on your sliced avocado and seal your meal tightly to prevent excess air from getting in.

4. Prep your soups. You'll be prepping and refrigerating (or freezing) three servings of soup for each recipe.

- For Nikki's Thai Sweet Potato Soup:
  - Review the recipe.
  - Chop the sweet potatoes, cilantro, ginger, and cauliflower. Crush the garlic. Add these ingredients to a soup pot, then follow steps 2 to 4 of the recipe.
  - Divide the soup into three freezable, microwaveable containers. Freeze or refrigerate.

- For the Broccoli Soup with Quinoa and Cilantro Sauce:
  - Review the recipe.
  - Chop the broccoli, leek, carrot, mushroom stems, and parsley (reserve some parsley for garnishing) and follow steps 1 to 3 of the recipe.
  - Add quinoa to the bottoms of three freezable, microwaveable containers. Portion the soup among the three containers. Freeze or refrigerate.
  - Prepare the dressing and refrigerate.

5. Prep your stir-fry. You'll be prepping one serving.

- For the Sensational Stir-Fry:
  - Review the recipe.
  - Chop the broccoli, onion, mushroom, and basil. Slice the yellow, orange, or red bell pepper. Place this veggie mixture in a baggie or container along with the quinoa and refrigerate.
  - Prep the sauce and refrigerate.
  - All your ingredients are now ready for the stir-fry. All you have to do is sauté them in a wok or saucepan.

6. Clean up. If you clean up as you go, you'll save time in the end.

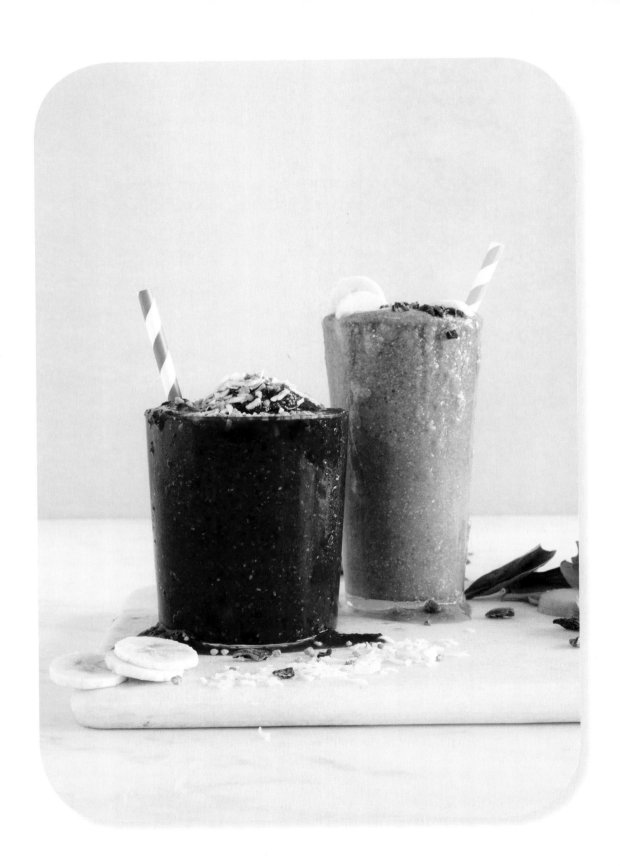

Breakfasts

Super Meal Smoothie

Makes 3 servings for the week

This nourishing smoothie will kick-start your morning. If you want to mix it up, try swapping out the pineapple for cherries or a banana, using homemade almond milk instead of coconut water, and adding cinnamon or cardamom. When you're ready to drink the smoothie, try adding toppings such as coconut flakes, goji berries, bee pollen, or pomegranate seeds.

Ingredients
3 handfuls kale or spinach
¾-inch piece ginger, peeled
3 cups pineapple chunks, fresh or frozen
3 tablespoons chia seeds
3 tablespoons coconut oil
½ tablespoon spirulina powder (optional)
½ tablespoon wheatgrass powder (optional)
3 cups coconut water
Handful of crushed ice

Directions
1. Add all ingredients to your blender and blend until smooth.
2. If the smoothie is too thick, add a small bit of water or more coconut water until desired consistency is reached; otherwise, omit some liquid to keep it thicker.
3. When consuming, add optional toppings such as unsweetened coconut flakes, bee pollen, goji berries, or pomegranate seeds.

Ginger Beet Smoothie

Makes 3 servings for the week

This is one of my absolute favorite smoothies. Beets help oxygenate your blood, flush your liver, and give you glowing skin, and I love pairing them with cucumbers, which are very hydrating. By adding ginger and lemon to this recipe, as well as a pinch of turmeric, you've created a super meal that will satisfy you, increase your energy levels, and banish cravings.

Ingredients
6-inch piece cucumber
1 large beet, peeled
1 ½ frozen bananas
¾ cup frozen cherries
2 cups water
3 tablespoons chia seeds
¾ inch ginger, chopped
3 tablespoons coconut oil
Juice of 1 lemon
1 tablespoon maca powder
½ tablespoon turmeric powder
Handful of crushed ice

Directions
1. Roughly chop the fruits and vegetables. Add all ingredients to a blender and blend until smooth.
2. If the smoothie is too thick, add a small bit of water until desired consistency is reached.

Lunches

Pomegranate-Arugula Salad

Makes 3 servings for the week

Salads are one of my favorite meals to prep and bring to work with me because they're so incredibly versatile. You can play with different flavors, textures, and colors. The key to making a great salad? Make sure to have three or more colors in the mix. Use different salad dressings, add steamed or roasted vegetables, or keep it fully raw. Or swap out quinoa for steamed edamame. There are so many ways to make a salad uber-delicious.

Other ways to add variety: use black beans instead of quinoa; skip the cucumber and use chopped carrots instead; try radishes instead of pomegranate seeds.

Note: To make meal prep as easy as possible, following the recipe is key. I would advise following each recipe as written for one week and seeing how it goes. Once you get the knack of meal prep, you can start to mix and match different ingredients.

Ingredients
3 large handfuls arugula
3-inch piece cucumber, finely diced
¾ cup cherry tomatoes, sliced in half
3 tablespoons pomegranate seeds
1 ½ cups cooked buckwheat groats
1 fennel bulb, diced
1 avocado, sliced, or 3 tablespoons toasted pumpkin seeds
3 handfuls cilantro, chopped
3 leaves red cabbage, finely chopped
3 tablespoons pumpkin seeds (optional)
Salad dressing of choice (pages 251–253)

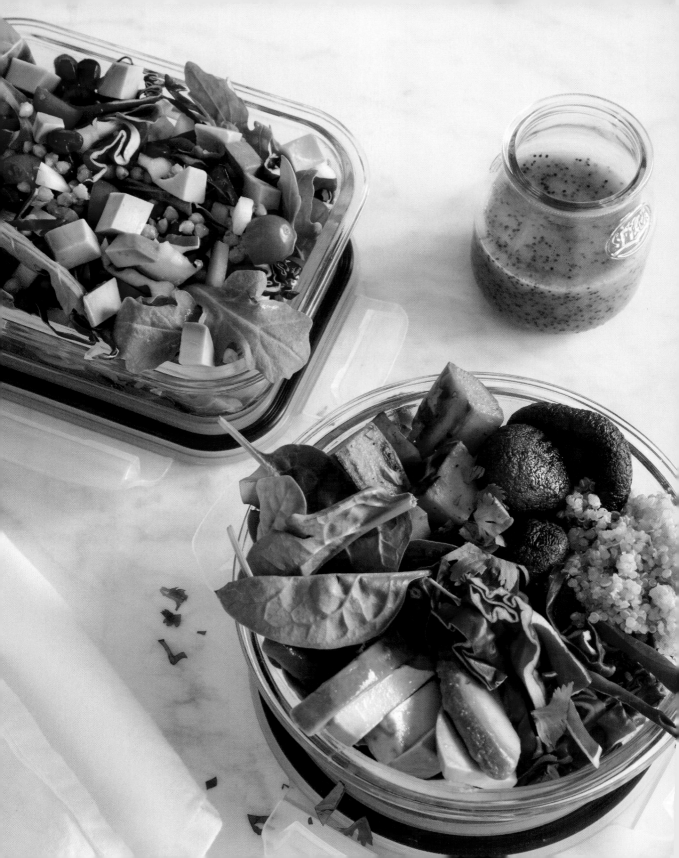

Directions

1. Divide all ingredients except the dressing between 3 separate bowls or plastic containers, or layer in 3 mason jars. (All your ingredients will already be prepped, so there won't be any cooking or chopping unless you choose to chop ingredients each day to preserve the freshness of the vegetables.) Refrigerate.

2. If using the pumpkin seeds in this recipe, toast them by heating a pan on medium heat until warm. Add pumpkin seeds, allow them to warm for 30 seconds, then shake the pan to mix them up. Continue until the seeds begin to puff up, around 4 to 5 minutes. Remove before they brown.

3. Add dressing to the salad just before you eat it, to preserve the crispness of the greens.

HOW TO PREP FENNEL

Fennel is an amazing food, but a lot of people don't know how to prep it. Here are some easy steps:

Step 1: Wash the fennel. Cut off the stalks where they meet the top of the bulb. Don't just throw the stalks out, though: they can be used to flavor stocks and soups. The leftover stalks can be minced and tossed into a salad or sauce, or used as a garnish.

Step 2: Trim off the root end.

Step 3: Stand the bulb on the root end and slice through it lengthwise.

Step 4: Using the tip of your knife, remove the core, which is the solid white piece at the root end of the bulb.

Step 5: Turn the bulb flat-side down so the striations are oriented top to bottom and slice into thin strips. If you want larger wedges (for roasting), simply cut each half into 3 to 4 pieces as desired. If you want to dice it, slice it into tiny pieces.

A prep pointer: Sliced fennel will brown (like a cut apple). If you're not going to use it right away, add the pieces to a bowl of cold water with half of a lemon squeezed in. The acid in the lemon juice will help prevent the oxidation that causes browning. (Hint: This works great for apple slices too!) You can store the fennel like this at room temperature for several hours or in the fridge, covered, overnight.

Buddha Bowl

Makes 4 servings for the week

The unusual name, Buddha Bowl, describes a salad-type dish that is packed so full it looks like the rounded belly of Buddha. It can be served hot or cold, and will taste delicious both ways.

The key to making the Buddha Bowl is to have all your ingredients already prepped: your potatoes should be roasted, your quinoa cooked, and vegetables chopped. Then you just add all the ingredients to your bowl, which takes only a minute or two.

I can eat the same bowl a few days in a row, but if you want more variety, switch up some of the ingredients on day two or three. Try swapping out quinoa for chickpeas or black beans, or use tomatoes instead of cabbage. Another option is to use all roasted vegetables on one day, and raw vegetables on another day. The goal is to start mixing and matching ingredients that you already have meal prepped, so that you never get bored.

Ingredients
3 sweet potatoes
2 pounds cremini mushrooms, or mushroom of choice
3 to 4 tablespoons olive oil
Salt and pepper
4 tablespoons liquid aminos
4 cups spinach
1 cup cooked quinoa
4 to 6 leaves red cabbage, finely chopped
1 avocado
2 handfuls chopped basil
Pinch cayenne (optional)
Pinch turmeric powder (optional)

Directions

1. Preheat the oven to 425 degrees.

2. Cut the sweet potatoes into roughly equal-sized cubes and place on a parchment-lined baking sheet.

3. Wash the cremini mushrooms and remove the stems. (Save the stems to be used in Broccoli Soup with Quinoa and Cilantro Sauce.) Place the caps of the mushrooms on another parchment-lined tray. You want to make sure that both the sweet potatoes and mushrooms are not overcrowded, otherwise they will not roast properly.

4. Drizzle half the olive oil on the sweet potatoes, along with a pinch of salt and pepper. Use the remaining olive oil on the mushrooms, along with the liquid aminos.

5. After 15 minutes, check the mushrooms and remove if they are tender and juicy. Toss the sweet potatoes and roast for another few minutes until they are crisp on the outside. Set the mushrooms and sweet potatoes aside.

6. Divide the spinach among four separate bowls, keeping the bowls in one area. Add the mushrooms next, then the sweet potatoes, then the quinoa mixture, followed by the cabbage and avocado—all evenly divided among four portions. Top with basil. Cover and refrigerate.

7. When ready to serve, add cayenne or turmeric and your dressing of choice.

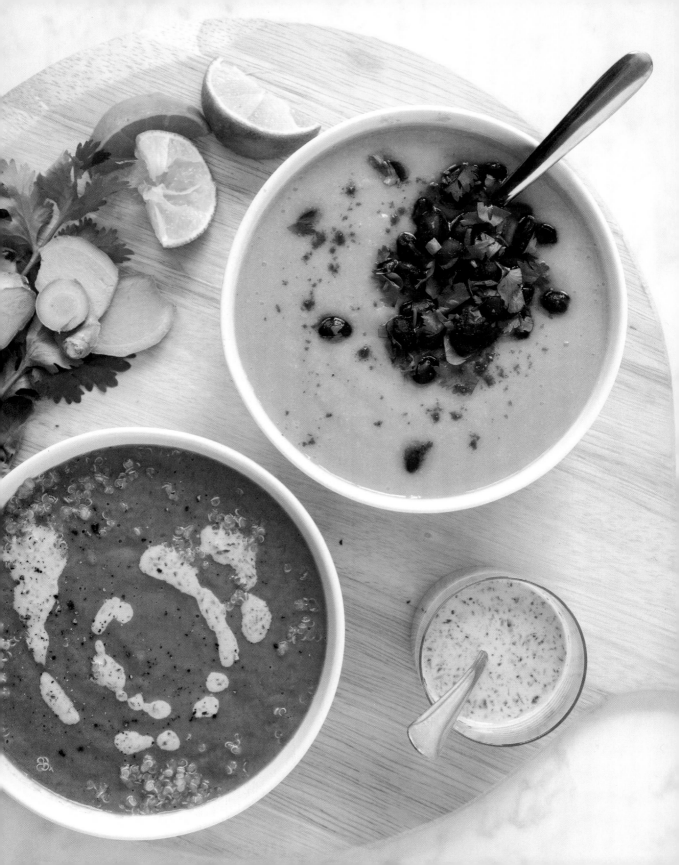

Dinners

Nikki's Thai Sweet Potato Soup

Makes 3 servings for the week

Thai food is one of my favorite cuisines because I love all the different flavors. I did a chef training course in Thailand, so I can confidently say that this vegan version won't fail your taste buds! If you're feeling adventurous, you can add lemongrass and a bay leaf to the stock (remove before you blend) for extra flavor and nutritional benefits. This soup does make a bit of extra, depending on how large your bowl is; however, soup freezes beautifully. You can add ¼ cup cooked black beans, ¼ cup cooked quinoa, extra veggies, or ¼ cup chopped cooked chicken if you like.

Ingredients
1 tablespoon olive oil
3 cloves garlic, crushed
¾ onion, roughly chopped
1 ½-inch piece ginger, peeled and chopped
1 can full-fat coconut milk
2 cups vegetable stock
2 sweet potatoes, washed and cubed
1 large head cauliflower, chopped into florets
Juice of 2 limes
Zest of 1 lime
1 handful cilantro, chopped
1 tablespoon black pepper
2 tablespoons turmeric powder

Directions
1. Heat the oil in a large pot over medium-high heat. Add garlic, onion, and ginger and cook until the onion is translucent.

145

2. Add coconut milk, vegetable stock, and sweet potatoes. Cover and bring to a boil. Once boiling, reduce to a simmer and cook for 5 minutes, covered.

3. Add the chopped cauliflower to the pot, along with the lime juice and zest. Cover and allow to simmer until the cauliflower is soft, about 5 more minutes. Add cilantro, pepper, and turmeric.

4. If using a blender, transfer the liquid to the blender container and blend until smooth; otherwise use a handheld immersion blender. You can blend the mixture until fully smooth or leave it slightly chunky, whatever you prefer. If the mixture is too thick, blend in a small bit of vegetable stock until the desired consistency is reached. Add salt and pepper to taste.

5. Divide among three bowls. Cover and refrigerate.

Broccoli Soup with Quinoa and Cilantro Sauce

Makes 3 servings for the week

I grew up eating my mom's fabulous broccoli soup, so this recipe is an homage to her! I like to blend it until it's not quite smooth, leaving some vegetable chunks for texture. You can also swap out the quinoa for any of the super grains to change it up—all of them will be great.

Ingredients
1 tablespoon olive oil
2 garlic cloves, crushed
1 teaspoon ground cumin
1 small onion, finely diced
1 firm white leek, green tops chopped off
Cremini mushroom stems, roughly chopped (saved from Buddha Bowl prep)
2 small heads of broccoli, roughly chopped
2 celery stalks, finely diced
1 carrot, peeled and finely chopped
1 tablespoon miso
1 cup vegetable stock
1 can full-fat coconut milk
1 cup kale or spinach

1 small handful parsley, chopped
¾ cup quinoa, cooked, and divided
Cilantro Tahini Dressing

Directions

1. In a large pot over medium-high heat, add olive oil along with crushed garlic, onion, chopped leek (discard the green top), cumin, and chopped mushroom stems until softened, around 3 minutes.

2. Add the broccoli, celery, carrot, miso, vegetable stock, and coconut milk, bringing the liquid to a boil. Reduce to a simmer, cover, and let cook 10 minutes.

3. Once the broccoli is soft, add the kale or spinach and the parsley. Cook until greens are soft, around 1 minute.

4. Blend the soup mixture, either in batches in a blender or in the pot with a handheld immersion blender, until smooth.

5. To serve, add ½ cup quinoa to the bottom of each of three bowls. Pour the soup into each of the bowls.

6. Cover each bowl and refrigerate.

7. When ready to serve, drizzle 1 tablespoon Cilantro Tahini Dressing (page 252) on top of each serving.

Sensational Stir-Fry

Makes 1 serving for the week

This stir-fry is quick to make and beyond satisfying. You eat it for dinner instead of lunch because it is better for your digestion to have cooked food at night—it gives your digestive system a rest, while still allowing you to absorb all the necessary nutrients.

Ingredients
¼ cup chopped broccoli
¼ cup sliced yellow, orange, or red bell pepper
¼ cup shelled edamame
1 tablespoon chopped onion
¼ portobello mushroom, chopped
Sensational Stir-Fry Sauce (recipe follows)
¼ cup cooked quinoa
Small handful basil, chopped

Directions
1. Heat a pan over high heat. Add ¼ cup water along with broccoli, bell pepper, edamame, onion, and mushroom. Stir-fry until vegetables are tender.
2. Once all the liquid has evaporated, add the sauce and quinoa and mix well.
3. Plate the stir-fry and sprinkle with chopped basil.

Sensational Stir-Fry Sauce

Ingredients
1 tablespoon tahini
½ tablespoon balsamic vinegar
1 teaspoon apple cider vinegar
Juice of ½ lime
¼ teaspoon black pepper
¼ teaspoon cayenne

Directions
1. Mix all the ingredients together.

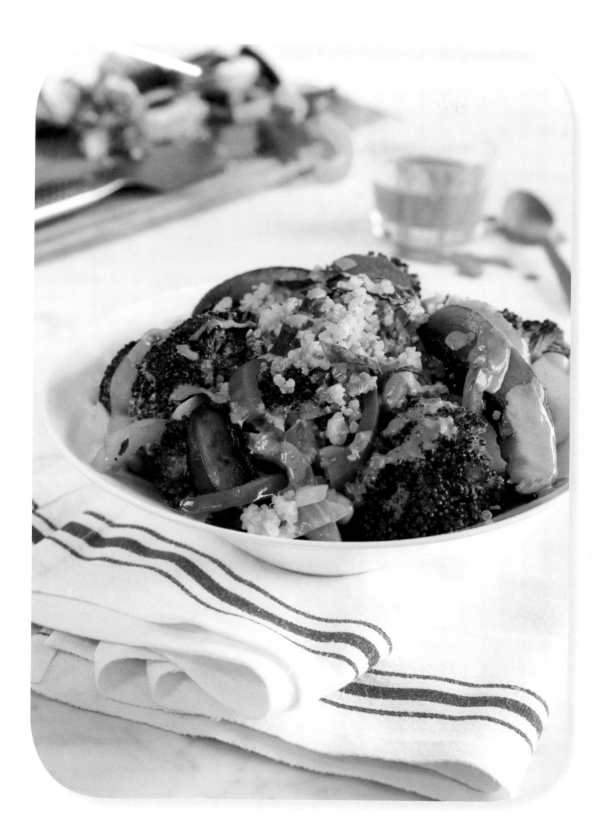

WEEK 2

<u>BREAKFASTS</u>:
- Vanilla Chia Pudding
- Chocolate Orange Smoothie
- Egg Veggie Millet

<u>LUNCHES</u>:
- Mason Jar Salad x3
- Noodles & Cashew Cream
- Lettuce-on-the-GO ☺

<u>DINNERS</u>:
- Stuffed Peppers
- Miso Glazed Salmon/Tempeh
- Roasted Veg /Salad
- Stir Fry

What <u>dessert</u> would I like?
↳ Peanut butter cups

<u>Snacks</u> for the week:
- hummus & beet chips
- crunchy chickpeas

<u>TO-DO</u>:
1) Go shopping - Bring List
2) Look at timeline
3) Sunday -
4) Lin. -

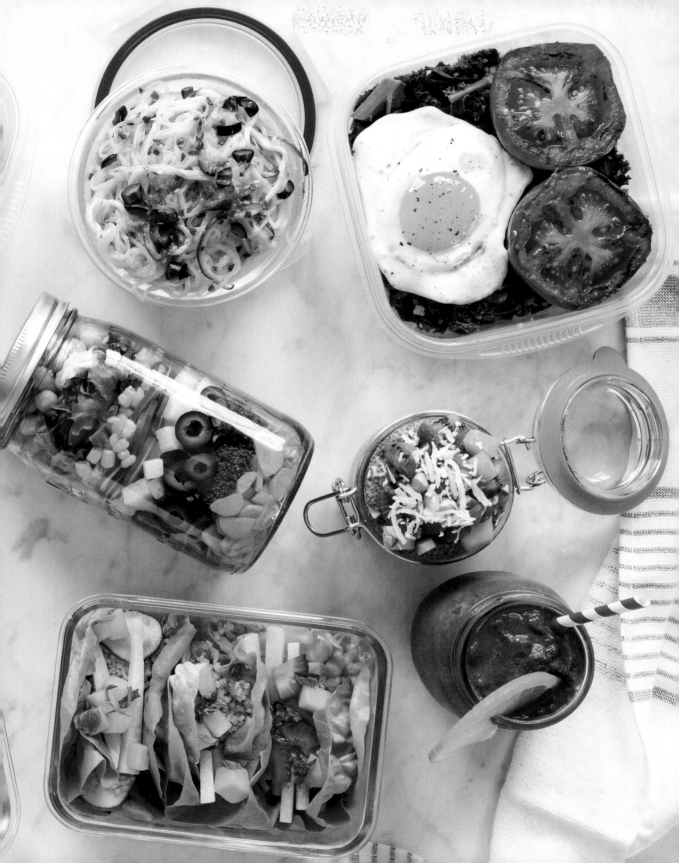

CHAPTER 12

Week Two—Fiber Up

Here's where you'll give your body a big-time fiber bump—with beans, corn, quinoa, millet, chia seeds, almonds, cashews, and more. Fiber has long been touted for its digestive and fat-fighting benefits, but new scientific research is also proclaiming fiber's ability to strengthen immune health and reduce the risk of obesity, type 2 diabetes, cardiovascular disease, and certain cancers.

Keep in mind the notes from week one regarding snacks; if you are feeling overwhelmed, either stick to the snacks you made in week one or plan on small handfuls of raw nuts, fresh fruit, or vegetables with hummus.

WEEK TWO MEAL PLAN

	Monday	Tuesday	Wednesday	Thursday	Friday	Saturday	Sunday
Breakfast	Vanilla Chia Pudding	Vanilla Chia Pudding	Vanilla Chia Pudding	Chocolate Orange Smoothie	Chocolate Orange Smoothie	Egg, Veggie, Millet	Egg, Veggie, Millet
Lunch	Mason Jar Salad	Mason Jar Salad	Mason Jar Salad	Noodles and Cashew Cream	Noodles and Cashew Cream	Lettuce-on-the-Go	Lettuce-on-the-Go
Dinner	Stuffed Red Peppers	Stuffed Red Peppers	Miso-Glazed Salmon or Tempeh	Roasted Vegetables over Salad	Roasted Vegetables over Salad	Roasted Vegetables over Salad	Sensational Stir-Fry

Snacks: Choose 1–2 per day from pages 237–249

Grocery List for Week Two

Vegetables

Avocado, 1

Basil, 1 small package

Bell pepper, 2 red, 1 any color

Broccoli florets, 2 cups

Butter lettuce, 1 head

Carrots, 5

Jicama, 1

Kale, 16-ounce package

Mint, 1 small package

Mixed greens, 16-ounce package

Onion, 1 small

Radishes, 12

Portobello mushroom, 1

Spinach, 16-ounce package

Tomato, 5

Zucchini, 1

2 pounds various veggies for roasting: potato, beet, butternut squash, asparagus, mushrooms, Brussels sprouts, or any other desired vegetables

Fruits

Banana, 1

Kiwi, 1

Lemon, 1

Limes, 2

Mango, 2

Medjool dates, 1 small carton

Oranges, 2

Grains

Millet, 16-ounce package

Quinoa (if you have none left over from the previous week)

Additional

Black beans, 15-ounce can

Black olives, pitted, 6-ounce can

Cashews, raw, ½ cup

Corn, 15-ounce can

Eggs, 2

Kelp noodles, 12-ounce package

Nut milk, 1 carton or 5 cups homemade

Salmon, wild-caught, 1 fillet

Tempeh, 1 8-ounce package

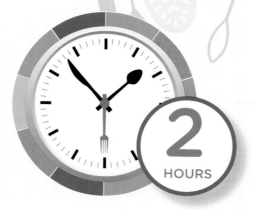

Overview:
Meal Prep Timing—Week Two

5 minutes: Prepare area

30 minutes: Prep breakfasts

20 minutes: Prep salads

20 minutes: Prep Noodles and Cashew Cream

15 minutes: Prep Stuffed Red Peppers

15 minutes: Prep Sensational Stir-Fry

< 2 hours: total time*

* With optional snacks: Add 10 to 45 minutes to the total time

Meal Prep for Week Two

1. Several recipes this week call for cooked grains and soaked nuts, and this part of prepping takes some ahead-of-time work. Cook enough quinoa to yield 1½ cups (for Lettuce-on-the-Go and Stuffed Red Peppers); enough buckwheat groats to yield 1 cup (for Roasted Veggies over Salad); and enough cooked millet to yield ½ cup (for Super Brekki). Also, soak raw cashews for at least 8 hours (for the Noodles and Cashew Cream). You'll also need 3 cups of nut milk such as almond milk, so you'll want to prep that ahead of time, too. See the nut milk instructions on page 117.

2. Clear your area to make sure you have plenty of room for prepping. Gather together all your gadgets, cutlery, utensils, cookware, and containers.

3. Prep your breakfasts.

   - For the Vanilla Chia Pudding: You'll be prepping three servings.

     - Review the recipe.

     - If using homemade nut milk, follow recipe on page 117 on making your own.

     - Follow step 1 and portion the mixture into three separate containers. Seal well and refrigerate.

     - Chop the fruit and place in separate baggies. Refrigerate.

     - Prior to serving, top the pudding with fruit and suggested toppings.

   - For the Chocolate Orange Smoothie: You'll be prepping two servings.

     - Review the recipe.

     - In each baggie, place spinach, banana, orange, chia seeds, dates, cacao powder, maca powder, and baobab. Seal each baggie and freeze.

- When you're ready for your smoothie, place the frozen ingredients in the blender. Add almond milk and vanilla extract. Blend well and serve.

- For the Egg, Veggie, and Millet: You'll be prepping two servings.

  - Review the recipe.

  - Cut the tomato in half. Place in a baggie and refrigerate. Chop the basil. Place it in a separate baggie and refrigerate.

  - Cook the millet according to package directions or see instructions on page 95). You'll need ½ cup cooked grain.

  - Follow steps 1 and 2 when you're ready to enjoy this breakfast.

4. Prep your lunches.

- For the Mason Jar Salad: You'll be prepping three salads, so you'll need three mason jars.

  - Review the recipe.

  - Chop the carrots and jicama. Slice tomatoes and radishes. Set each prepped veggie aside separately.

  - Steam the broccoli until just tender. Then chop it and set aside to cool.

  - Layer the ingredients in the jars, as directed, beginning with 2 tablespoons salad dressing. Refrigerate until ready to serve.

- For the Noodles and Cashew Cream: You'll be prepping two servings.

  - Review the recipe.

  - The cashews will need to soak for 8 hours, so you might want to do this first thing in the morning of your prep day. After 8 hours, drain and rinse.

- Boil the kelp noodles, as directed.

- While noodles are cooking, spiralize the zucchini and set aside.

- Prep the sauce: In a blender or food processor, blend together pre-soaked cashews, water, liquid aminos, nutritional yeast flakes, and spices. Set aside.

- Drain the kelp noodles and add spiralized zucchini. Mix well. Stir in sauce.

- Divide the dish into two containers. Refrigerate.

- For the Lettuce-on-the-Go: You'll be prepping two servings.

  - Review the recipe.

  - Chop your mango, jicama, strawberries, and radish. Place into separate containers or on a chopping board.

  - Prep quinoa according to package directions or see instructions on page 96. Put cooked quinoa and toasted pumpkin seeds into other bowls or containers.

  - Add equal amounts of each ingredient into your butter lettuce cups. Drizzle with dressing of choice and top with chopped mint.

  - Place cups into two containers, seal and then refrigerate.

5. Prep your dinners.

- For the Stuffed Red Peppers: You'll be prepping two servings.

  - Review the recipe.

  - Mix together the ingredients for the stuffing. Cut peppers in half.

  - Fill the pepper halves with the stuffing mixture and bake.

  - Place the stuffed peppers in a container, cover, and refrigerate.

- Reheat in the microwave when you're ready to serve it or reheat in the oven under the broiler for a few minutes.

- For the Miso-Glazed Salmon or Tempeh, you'll be prepping one serving.

  - Review the recipe.

  - Bake this ahead of time and refrigerate, so you can reheat later, if desired.

  - Serve with your choice of salad or extra roasted vegetables topped with the extra miso dressing.

- For the Roasted Vegetables over Salad, you'll be prepping three servings.

  - Review the recipe.

  - Decide which vegetables you will be roasting and check the roasting chart on page 39 for cook times depending on vegetable.

  - Prepare other parts of the recipe. Then divide into containers.

- For the Sensational Stir-Fry, you'll be prepping one serving.

  - Review the recipe.

  - Chop all vegetables: broccoli, bell pepper, onion, and portobello mushroom.

  - Prepare the sauce. Set aside.

  - Cook the vegetables.

  - Mix together the veggies, quinoa, and sauce. Place in a container. Seal well and refrigerate. Make sure you have prepped quinoa according to package directions or instructions on page 96.

  - Reheat and garnish with chopped basil.

6. Clean up. If you clean up as you go, you'll save time in the end.

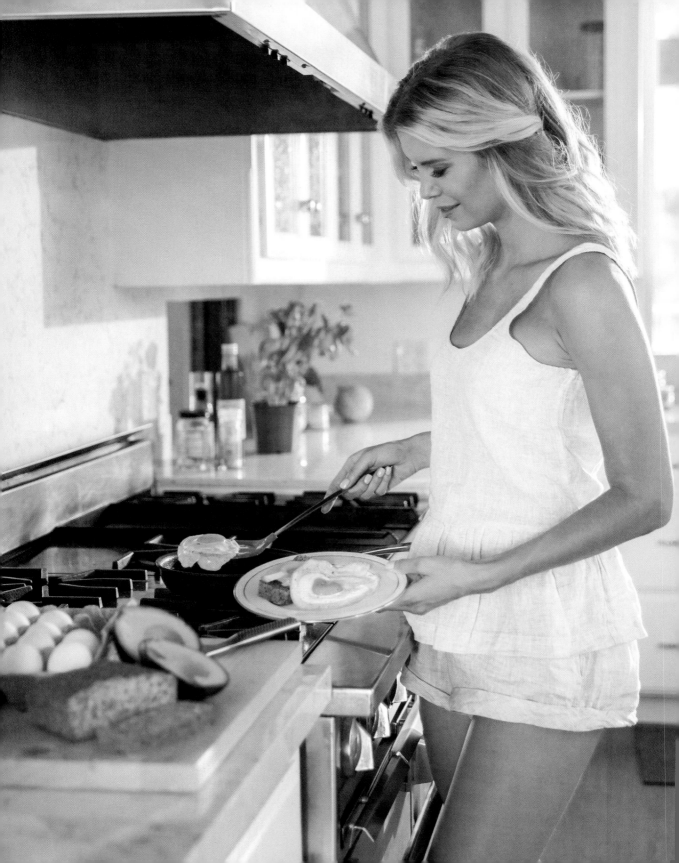

Breakfasts

Vanilla Chia Pudding

Makes 3 servings for the week

Here's a near-perfect prep breakfast—you quickly mix together several ingredients, store in the fridge overnight, and enjoy in the morning. Voilà! I recommend using homemade almond or another nut milk, which you can find on page 119. Alternatively, you can use store bought almond, rice, or coconut milk. The fruits can be swapped out according to preference.

Ingredients
¾ cup chia seeds
3 cups nut milk of choice
2 teaspoons cinnamon, plus more for topping
1 teaspoon vanilla extract
6 mint leaves, finely chopped
1 cup chopped mango and kiwi
3 tablespoons slivered or sliced almonds
2 tablespoons coconut flakes
1 tablespoon bee pollen (optional)
1 tablespoon goji berries (optional)

Directions
1. Mix the chia seeds, nut milk, cinnamon, vanilla, and mint in a bowl, then divide among three containers or mason jars. Allow the mixture to sit for at least an hour, and preferably overnight, for the mixture to thicken. If mixture becomes too thick, add a small amount of water and stir.
2. When you're ready to eat, add your pre-portioned fruit and top with

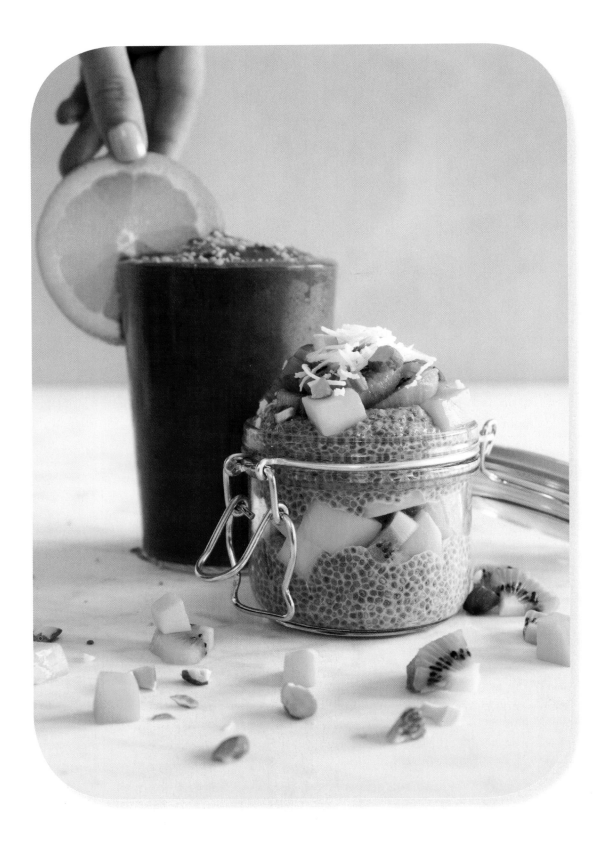

chopped or sliced almonds, coconut flakes, and extra cinnamon. Add bee pollen and goji berries to the topping, if using.

Chocolate Orange Smoothie

Makes 2 servings for the week

I love this smoothie because it tastes so different from others you may have had. Orange and chocolate are a great combination, and it's a decadent yet healthy way to start your day. If you'd like the orange flavor to be more intense, add the zest of one of the oranges.

Ingredients
2 handfuls spinach
1 ½ cups almond milk
1 frozen banana
2 oranges, peeled and seeds removed
2 tablespoons chia seeds
4 Medjool dates, pitted
3 tablespoons raw cacao powder
1 teaspoon vanilla extract
2 teaspoons maca powder
2 teaspoons baobab
1 teaspoon cacao nibs (optional)
1 teaspoon coconut flakes (optional)
1 teaspoon bee pollen (optional)

Directions
1. Put all ingredients except cacao nibs, coconut flakes, and pollen into a blender with a handful of ice. Blend until smooth. If the mixture is too thick, add a small amount of water.
2. Divide between two small mason jars and top each with raw cacao nibs, coconut flakes, and bee pollen.

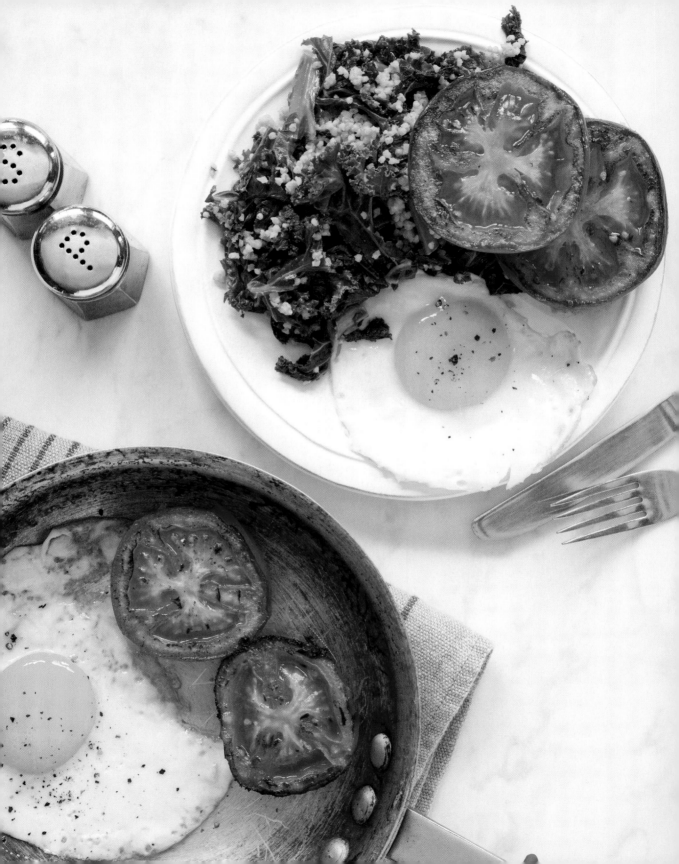

Super Brekkie

Makes 2 servings for the week

Millet is a versatile, quick-cooking, gluten-free whole grain that's loaded with protein, fiber, and nutrients. And it's more economical than quinoa—which is great for the budget-conscious. This recipe is a true super meal, thanks not only to millet but also to its companion foods: kale, tomato, basil, turmeric, and cayenne.

Ingredients
4 teaspoons olive oil
2 cups kale
½ cup cooked millet
2 dashes liquid aminos
1 teaspoon turmeric powder
¼ teaspoon cayenne
2 eggs
2 tomatoes, cut in half
Salt and pepper
Small handful basil, chopped

Directions
1. Heat a pan on medium heat and add 2 teaspoons olive oil. After a minute, add the kale. Once it's almost cooked, add the millet, liquid aminos, turmeric, and cayenne, stirring to combine. Transfer to a bowl.

2. In the same pan, add the remaining 2 teaspoons olive oil, distributing evenly. Add eggs to one side of the pan, the tomatoes cut-side down to the other. Season with salt and pepper. I like to switch it up between scrambled and sunny-side up, which is pictured. Cover and cook for 2 minutes. Once the eggs have begun to lightly crisp on the outside, carefully remove and divide between two separate bowls, along with the millet and kale. Using the spatula, carefully remove the tomatoes and add to your containers. Top with basil.

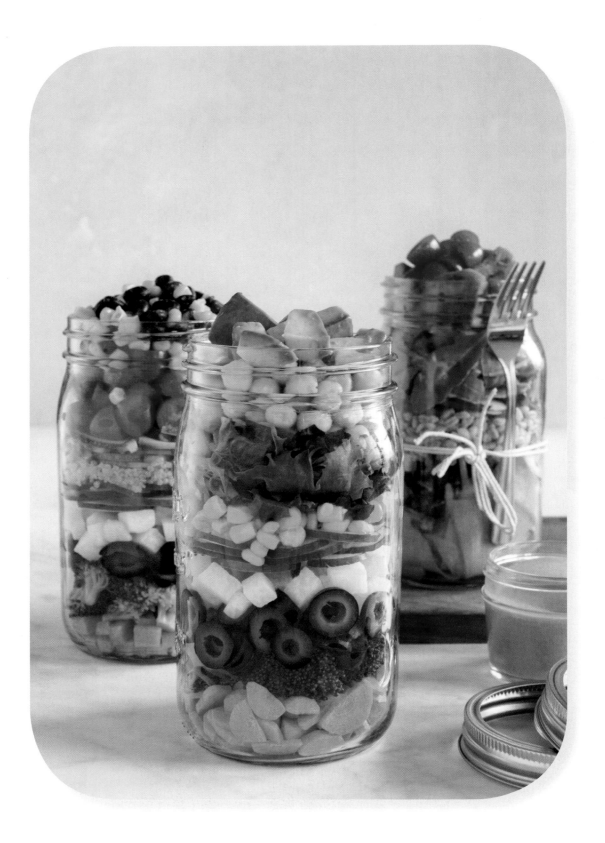

Lunches

Mason Jar Salad

Makes 3 servings for the week

I want you to get creative here! When making your salads over the next three days, choose different ingredients, change out the dressings, try dicing your vegetables or shredding them instead of slicing. Have fun, and don't forget that it's not about following the recipe to a T—it's about experimenting with new ingredients.

Ingredients
3 to 6 tablespoons salad dressing of choice (pages 251–253)
3 large carrots, peeled and sliced
6 radishes, sliced
15 black olives, sliced (optional)
¾ cup corn
¾ cup chopped steamed broccoli
¾ cup cooked black beans
3 tomatoes, sliced
3 tablespoons chopped jicama
1 avocado, sliced
3 handfuls mixed greens

Directions
1. Divide the dressing among three mason jars, adding to the bottom.
2. Next, divide the carrot, radishes, olives, corn, broccoli, black beans, tomatoes, jicama, and avocado, followed by the greens, among the jars. It doesn't necessarily need to go in this order; however, putting the greens on top helps to keep them from wilting.

HOW TO MEAL PREP JICAMA

To prep jicama, cut a thin slice off the top and bottom to create a flat surface. Begin from the top to bottom, and slide your knife under the skin to peel, following the curve. Continue around the whole way, using a vegetable peeler to get any tough skin off.

Make vertical cuts, creating slabs about ½-inch thick. Turn each slab onto its side and make more vertical cuts, until you have thin slices. You can also shred it or use a mandoline to create very thin matchsticks.

Jicama makes an excellent salsa. Simply dice it finely, and combine it with diced tomato, black beans, red onions, cilantro, and lime juice. It also complements ceviche beautifully, and can be turned into "rice" for raw sushi.

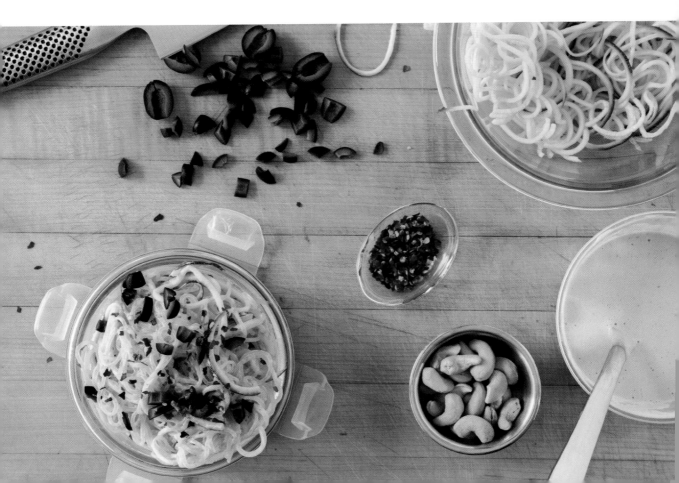

Noodles and Cashew Cream

Makes 2 servings for the week

This is an incredibly tasty alternative to pasta that will leave you wanting more. Feel free to add ¼ cup black beans, quinoa, some sautéed tempeh, or 2 tablespoons shredded chicken for extra protein. I also love to add shaved asparagus, chopped red pepper, and chopped basil. Or just eat it as is! It's a delicious meal either way.

Haven't heard of kelp noodles? Here's the lowdown: They're a low-calorie noodle made of kelp, a sea vegetable. They're naturally gluten-free, and high in calcium, iron, and vitamin K.

For a crunchy texture, add them uncooked to recipes. For a soft pasta-like texture, soak them in water with 1 tablespoon lemon juice or apple cider vinegar and a pinch of salt for 30 minutes.

Ingredients
Kelp noodles, 12-ounce package
1 tablespoon baking soda
½ cup raw cashews, soaked 8 hours
1 teaspoon lemon juice
1 teaspoon liquid aminos
1 tablespoon nutritional yeast flakes
¼ teaspoon paprika
1 zucchini

Directions
1. Rinse and drain the kelp noodles, then add to a bowl with hot water to cover and the baking soda. Let them sit for 20 minutes until they begin to soften.
2. While the noodles are soaking, drain the cashews and add to a blender along with ½ cup water, lemon juice, liquid aminos, nutritional yeast flakes, and paprika. Season with salt and pepper. Blend until smooth, scraping down sides of blender as necessary.
3. Cut the top and bottom off the zucchini, then use a spiralizer to create

noodles. If you don't have a spiralizer, use a peeler to create long thin strips.

4. Drain the kelp noodles. Add them to the bowl of zucchini noodles. Pour in the sauce and use your hands to mix the sauce into the noodles well. The longer the sauce sits on the noodles, the softer both the kelp and zucchini will become.

5. Divide between two containers and refrigerate.

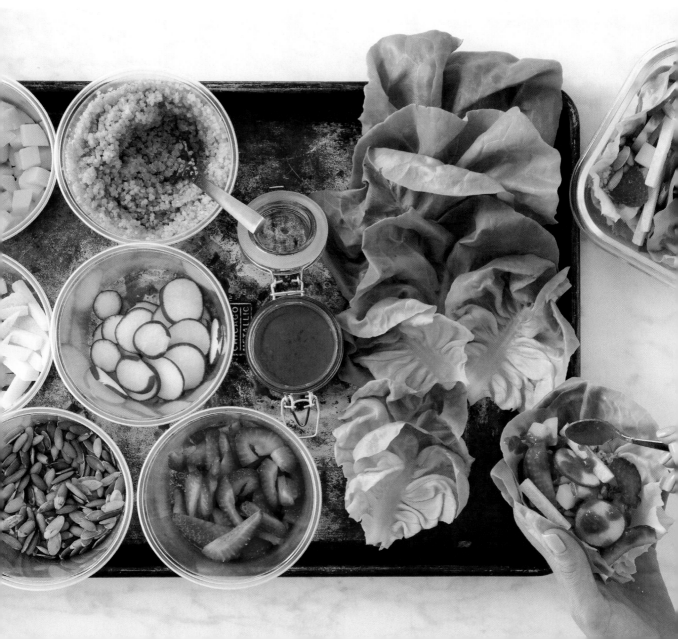

Lettuce-on-the-Go

Makes 2 servings for the week

After testing this recipe, which was originally supposed to be a salad, I realized that it was even more satisfying when turned into lettuce cups. All I can say is that Lettuce-on-the-Go is incredibly light, refreshing, and a satiating meal! You can choose to make smaller cups, which will use more leaves, or fill them up, leaving some of the butter lettuce for another meal.

Ingredients
1 head butter lettuce
2 tablespoons toasted pumpkin seeds
½ cup cooked quinoa
6 radishes, sliced
6 strawberries, sliced
12 mint leaves, finely chopped
½ cup jicama strips
½ mango, roughly chopped
Dressing of choice (pages 251–253), 1 to 2 tablespoons

Directions
1. Cut out the stem of the lettuce and separate the leaves, which will be the lettuce cups. Wash and spread them out on a chopping board in order to fill.
2. To toast the pumpkin seeds, add the seeds to a pan and turn the heat on medium. Cook for 2 minutes, rotating the pan so the seeds do not burn. Once they begin to expand and lightly brown, remove.
3. Divide the quinoa, radishes, strawberries, pumpkin seeds, mint, jicama, and mango among the lettuce cups. Top with dressing when ready to serve.
4. Portion the cups into two containers and refrigerate.

Dinners

Stuffed Red Peppers

Makes 2 servings for the week

This delicious dinner is packed with fiber. The beans give the recipe a meaty flavor, so if you've just started transitioning into plant-based eating, you'll love this meal. I like to add various vegetables, so feel free to follow the recipe exactly or add some chopped carrot and spinach, which are pictured in the photo. Cut the peppers however you like, either vertically or just cutting the tops off. Garnish with extra cilantro, an extra squeeze of lime, and any additional spices.

Ingredients
½ cup quinoa, cooked
½ cup black beans
¼ cup corn
1 large carrot, peeled and diced
Small handful spinach, roughly chopped
1 tablespoon finely diced onion
1 tablespoon nutritional yeast flakes
1 teaspoon ground cumin
Juice of 1 lime
1 tablespoon olive oil
Salt and pepper to taste
2 red bell peppers

Directions
1. Preheat the oven to 400 degrees and line a baking sheet with parchment paper.
2. In a bowl, mix the quinoa, black beans, corn, carrot, spinach, onion,

nutritional yeast flakes, cumin, lime juice, and olive oil. Season with salt and pepper.

3. Slice the peppers either vertically in half, removing the seeds and stem, or remove the tops and scoop out the seeds.

4. Divide the quinoa mixture between the peppers. Place in the oven and bake for 25 minutes.

5. Remove half the peppers, cool, and place in a container for the following night's dinner. To reheat, place under the broiler for 4 minutes.

Roasted Veggies over Salad

Makes 2 servings for the week

Roasted vegetables are some of my favorite things to make as an entree as well as a side dish or a topping for salads. I love using onions, potatoes, carrots, beets, butternut squash, Brussels sprouts, and other hearty root vegetables. Tender vegetables, such as asparagus and mushrooms, are also great veggies to use. This is a tasty meal that you can make easily, and it keeps very well for a few days.

Ingredients
2 tablespoons olive oil
2 cups roasted vegetables (see above for ideas)
2 platefuls arugula or other greens
1 cup cooked buckwheat groats or other super grain
Salad dressing of choice (pages 251–253)

Directions

1. Choose your vegetables according to preference and use the guide on page 39 to roast.

2. When ready to serve, place veggies over arugula and buckwheat groats. Mix with dressing of choice.

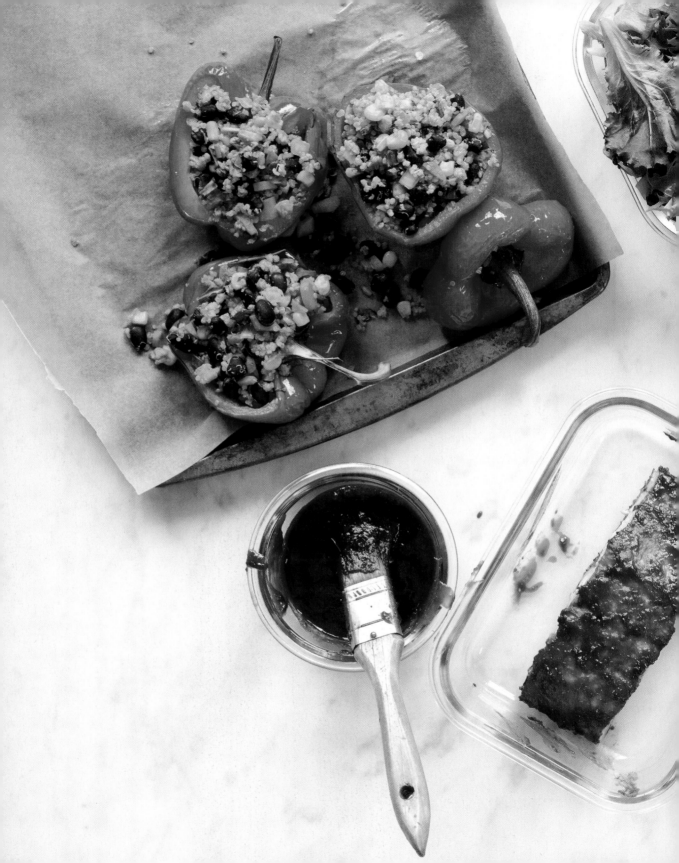

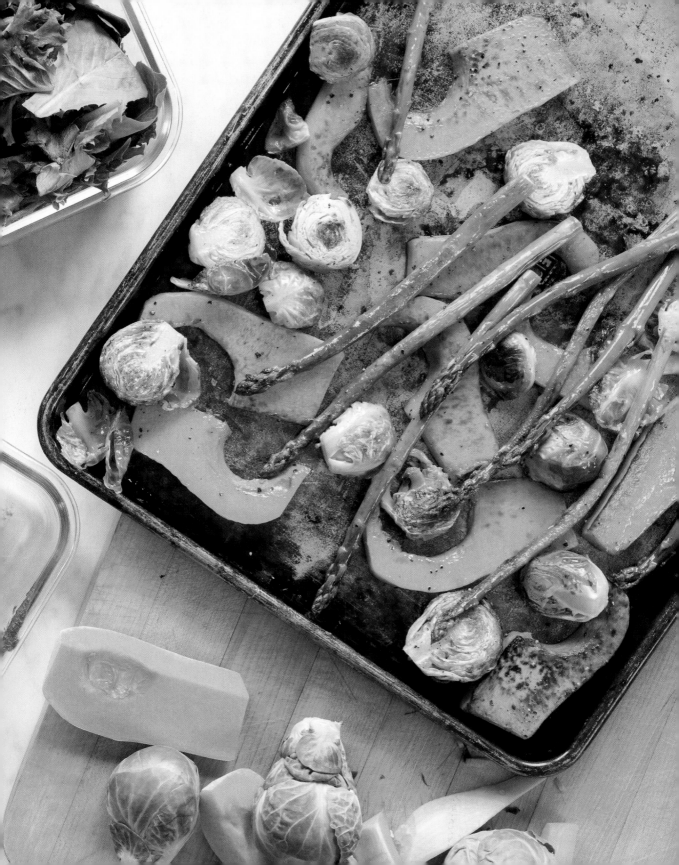

Miso-Glazed Salmon or Tempeh

Makes 1 serving for the week

I wanted to slip in a fish recipe because I realize that many people reading this are not eating a 100 percent plant-based diet. If you're in that group, I want to give you nutritious animal protein choices, so I selected salmon, one of the healthiest swimmers around. However, if you're vegan, simply replace the salmon with four slices of tempeh, around an inch thick. If you are choosing to do the salmon, I absolutely recommend buying wild-caught.

This meal is best served with a salad of your choice or any extra roasted vegetables you have. My favorite thing to do is add some greens, as well as some colorful vegetables such as tomatoes, carrots, jicama, or corn, then drizzle the extra miso dressing on top. Serve with your miso-glazed salmon or tempeh. This recipe is not calling for something specific as I'd like you to get creative and use what vegetables you have in the fridge that look appealing.

Ingredients
1 tablespoon olive oil
¼ cup white miso
1 tablespoon agave syrup
2 tablespoons reduced-sodium soy sauce
1 tablespoon grated ginger
4 ounces salmon fillet or 4 slices of tempeh

Directions
1. Preheat the oven to 400 degrees.
2. Coat a glass baking dish with olive oil.
3. In a small bowl, whisk together the miso, agave, soy sauce, and ginger. Reserve about a third of the mixture in a small bowl.
4. Place salmon skin-side down in the baking dish, or place the tempeh slices in the dish.

5. Brush the salmon or tempeh with the larger amount of miso mixture. Cover with plastic wrap and refrigerate for at least a half hour.

6. Remove the salmon or tempeh from the refrigerator and discard the plastic wrap. Bake the salmon or tempeh for 30 minutes, or until the fish flakes easily with a fork.

7. Transfer to plates and spoon the reserved miso sauce over the fish or tempeh. Serve with salad or roasted vegetables of choice.

Sensational Stir-Fry

(See page 148.)

Sensational Stir-Fry Sauce

(See page 148.)

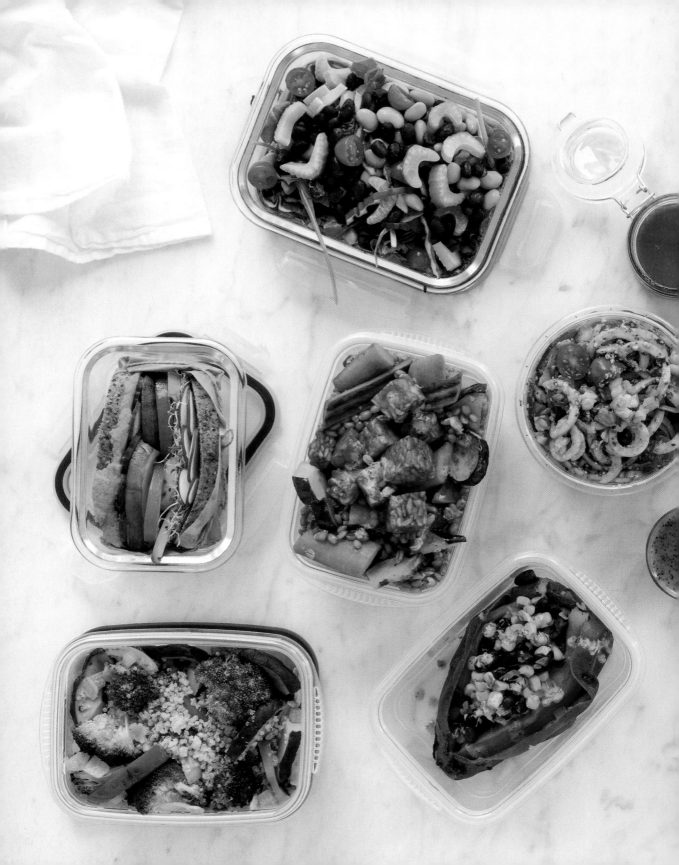

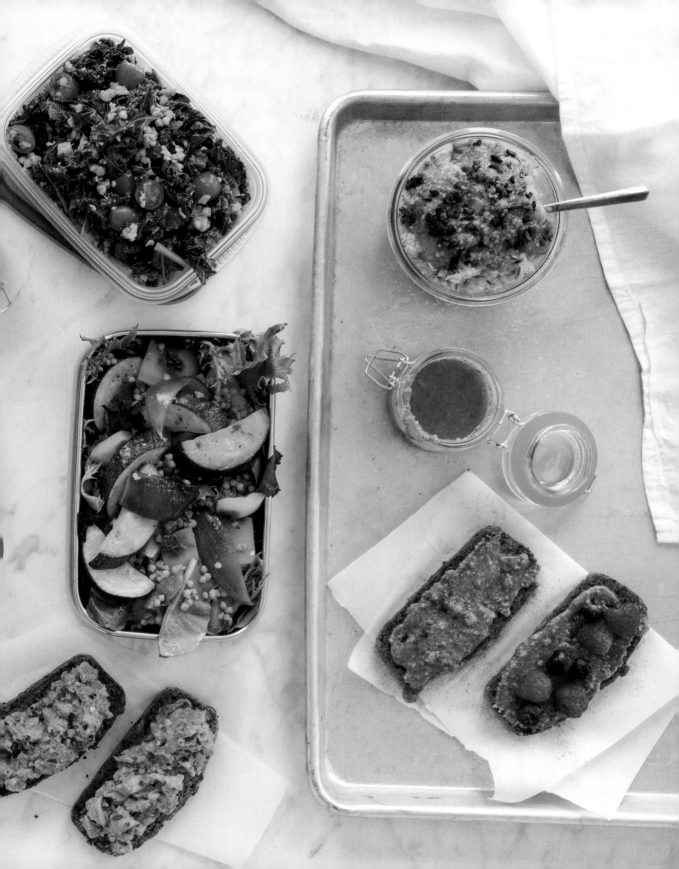

CHAPTER 13

Week Three—Protein Power

During week three, you'll bump up your protein intake to keep losing weight. As I mentioned earlier, protein helps maintain calorie-burning muscle, plus it keeps your metabolism running in high gear.

You'll be getting protein from foods such as edamame, hemp, and beans. Admittedly, these foods don't normally come to mind when you think of protein. But in the plant world, they're top protein sources—and are low in saturated fat, high in fiber, and cholesterol-free. An added bonus is that purchasing plant proteins helps keep your food costs lower.

WEEK THREE MEAL PLAN

	Monday	Tuesday	Wednesday	Thursday	Friday	Saturday	Sunday
Breakfast	Smashed Avocado on Toast	Smashed Avocado on Toast	Zoats with Maple Cinnamon Almond Butter	Zoats with Maple Cinnamon Almond Butter	Power Bowl	Power Bowl	Paleo Toast with Maple Cinnamon Almond Butter
Lunch	Salad with Edamame and Black Beans	Salad with Edamame and Black Beans	Salad with Edamame and Black Beans	Paleo Sandwich with Hummus	Paleo Sandwich with Hummus	Tri-Colored Salad	Tri-Colored Salad
Dinner	Zucchini Noodles with Hemp Pesto	Zucchini Noodles with Hemp Pesto	Loaded Mexican Baked Sweet Potato	Loaded Mexican Baked Sweet Potato	Roasted Vegetables with Spelt	Roasted Vegetables with Spelt	Sensational Stir-Fry

Grocery List for Week Three

Vegetables

Alfalfa sprouts, 1 small package

Arugula, two 16-ounce packages

Avocado, 2

Basil, 2 small packages

Bell pepper, any color

Broccoli, small bag of florets

Cherry tomatoes, 1–2 packages

Cilantro, 1 bunch

Cucumber, 1

Garlic, 1 bulb

Kale, 16-ounce package

Onion, 1 small

Portobello mushroom, 2

Red bell pepper, 1

Red cabbage, 1 small head

Shelled frozen edamame, 14-ounce package

Spinach, 16-ounce package

Sweet potatoes, 2

Tomato, 1

Zucchini, 5–6

Various types of veggies to roast: summer squash, onions, bell peppers, carrots, and so forth

Fruits

Berries, any type, 1 pint (or use strawberries leftover from previous week)

Lemon, 1

Limes, 4

Grains

Buckwheat groats, 16-ounce package

Oats, 18-ounce canister

Spelt berries, 24-ounce bag

Additional

Almonds, raw, 1 small package

Almond flour, 16-ounce package

Black beans, two 15-ounce cans

Chickpeas, 15-ounce can

Coconut flour, 16-ounce package

Corn, 15-ounce can

Eggs, 1 dozen

Tempeh, 11 slices

White wine vinegar, 17-ounce bottle

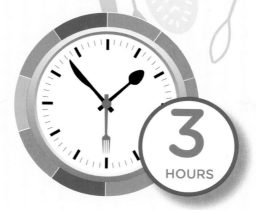

Overview:
Meal Prep Timing—Week Three

5 minutes: Prepare area

15 minutes: Prep and bake Paleo Bread

15 minutes: Chop vegetables for roasting; wrap 2 sweet potatoes in foil for baking

5 minutes: Prep the avocado mixture for the Smashed Avocado on Toast

15 minutes: Prep the Zoats

15 minutes: Prep the Maple Cinnamon Almond Butter

15 minutes: Prep the Power Bowl

20 minutes: Prep the Salad with Edamame and Black Beans

10 minutes: Prep the hummus

10 minutes: Prep the Tri-Colored Salad

20 minutes: Prep the Zucchini Noodles with Hemp Pesto

10 minutes: Prep the Loaded Mexican Baked Sweet Potato

10 minutes: Prep the Roasted Veggies over Salad

15 minutes: Prep the Sensational Stir-Fry

3 hours: total time*

*With optional snacks: Add 10 to 45 minutes to the total time

Meal Prep for Week Three

1. Several recipes this week call for baked bread (Paleo Bread) and cooked grains, and this part of prepping takes some ahead-of-time work. I suggest baking the bread first so that you have it on hand for the week. Cook enough quinoa to yield ¼ cup (for the Sensational Stir-Fry); enough buckwheat groats to yield 1 cup (for the Power Bowl); and enough spelt to yield 1 cup (for the Roasted Vegetables with Spelt). Please note too that spelt berries need to be soaked in water for 1 hour, or even overnight. Follow package directions or see instructions on page 96.

2. Clear your area to make sure you have plenty of room for prepping. Gather together all your gadgets, cutlery, utensils, cookware, and containers.

3. Wrap 2 sweet potatoes in foil and place on a baking sheet. Chop various veggies for roasting (around 5 cups raw).

4. Prep your breakfasts.

   - For the Smashed Avocado on Toast: You'll be prepping two servings.

     - Review the recipe.
     - Follow step 1 and portion the avocado mixture into two separate containers. Seal well and refrigerate.

   - For the Zoats: You'll be prepping two servings.

     - Review and prepare the recipe.
     - Portion the mixture into two separate containers. Seal well and refrigerate.

   - For the Maple Cinnamon Almond Butter: You'll be prepping a batch for the week.

     - Review the recipe.

- After blending all the ingredients together, place the butter in a sealed container or jar and refrigerate. The butter will last up to two weeks in the fridge.

- For the Power Bowl: You'll be prepping two servings.
  - Review the recipe.
  - Complete steps 1 and 2. Reserve the basil until you are ready to serve the dish.
  - Divide into two containers. Seal well and refrigerate.

- For the Paleo Toast with Maple Cinnamon Almond Butter: You'll be prepping one serving.
  - Review the recipe.
  - Toast your bread, spread almond butter, cinnamon, and berries. Seal well.

5. Prep your lunches.

- For the Salad with Edamame and Black Beans: You'll be prepping three salads.
  - Review the recipe.
  - Shred the cabbage, slice the celery, and chop the olives.
  - Combine all ingredients, reserving the salad dressing until ready to serve. You may want to portion the salad dressing into three small containers and refrigerate.
  - Portion the salads into three containers. Seal well and refrigerate.
  - Refrigerate until ready to serve.

- For the Paleo Sandwich with Hummus: You'll be prepping two servings.
  - Review the recipe.

- This sandwich can be assembled as needed and wrapped for work. You can prepare the hummus ahead of time. Roast the red pepper, as directed. Blend all the ingredients together. Place the hummus in a container. Seal well and refrigerate.

- For the Tri-Colored Salad: You'll be prepping two servings.

  - Review the recipe.

  - Chop your vegetables and divide between two containers, along with your arugula. Seal and refrigerate.

6. Prep your dinners.

- For the Zucchini Noodles with Hemp Pesto: You'll be prepping two servings.

  - Review the recipe.

  - Blend together all the pesto ingredients. Set aside.

  - Cook the tempeh.

  - While tempeh is cooking, spiralize zucchinis and place in two containers. Divide the sauce and add to each one, mixing well.

  - Add tomatoes and tempeh between both containers.

  - Seal and refrigerate.

- For the Loaded Mexican Baked Sweet Potato: You'll be prepping two servings.

  - Review the recipe.

  - Slice sweet potatoes in half, as directed. Bake.

  - While sweet potatoes are baking, chop garlic and onions. Sauté and set aside.

  - Add the black beans and corn to the garlic mixture.

  - Follow steps 4 and 5. Place each potato in a container. Seal and refrigerate.

- When ready to serve, reheat the dish and top with cilantro, lime juice, and salad dressing.

- For the Roasted Vegetables with Spelt: You'll be prepping two servings.
  - Review the recipe.
  - Divide the cooked spelt into two containers, and refrigerate.
  - Roast your vegetables according to preference and cook times on page 39.
  - Cook your tempeh and corn, then add to the spelt and roasted vegetables. Divide between two containers. Seal both containers well and refrigerate.

- For the Sensational Stir-Fry, you'll be prepping one serving.
  - Review the recipe.
  - Chop all vegetables: broccoli, bell pepper, onion, and portobello mushroom.
  - Cook quinoa. Set aside.
  - Prepare the sauce. Set aside.
  - Mix together the veggies, quinoa, and sauce. Place in a container. Seal well and refrigerate.
  - Reheat and garnish with chopped basil.

7. Clean up. If you clean up as you go, you'll save time in the end.

Breakfasts

Paleo Bread

Makes enough servings for the week, plus extra, which you can freeze

Not all breads are healthy, even though many companies would like you to believe so. The solution? Make your own! That way, you can monitor the ingredients that go into it, plus you know that it's gluten-free and thus easier on your digestive system. I love topping this bread with a few slices of avocado, turning it into sandwiches, or chopping up a piece or two and baking it into croutons for salad. I recommend you use a silicone loaf pan that's 8½ x 4½ inches. If you cannot find a silicone pan, opt for the tin version.

Ingredients
1 cup almond flour
¼ cup chia seeds
¼ cup ground flaxseed
¼ cup coconut flour
1 teaspoon baking soda
1 teaspoon xanthan gum
1 teaspoon salt
6 eggs
4 ½ tablespoons water
3 tablespoons white wine vinegar

Directions
1. Preheat the oven to 350 degrees.
2. Mix almond flour, chia seeds, flaxseed, coconut flour, baking soda, xanthan gum, and salt in a bowl.

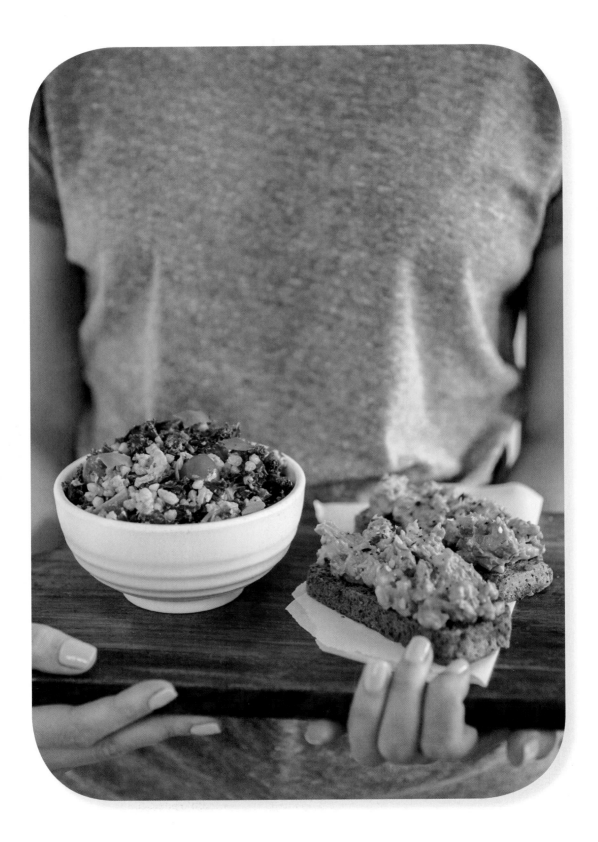

3. In a separate bowl, combine the eggs, water, and vinegar and mix well. Slowly pour the wet ingredients into the dry, mixing together as you pour.

4. Pour mixture into a coconut-oil-greased loaf pan and bake for 50 minutes. Remove from oven and allow to cool before taking the loaf out of the pan.

Maple Cinnamon Almond Butter

Makes enough for the week

Yes, you can make your own almond butter! It can seem a bit intimidating at first, but it's easy to do. Plus, I love knowing exactly what goes into it— no additives, preservatives, or salt, and not too much sugar. You'll save money too, since store-bought nut butters can be quite expensive.

Ingredients
¾ cup raw almonds
½ tablespoon cinnamon
1 tablespoon maca powder
1 tablespoon maple syrup
2 tablespoons coconut oil

Directions

1. In a high-speed blender or food processor, process the almonds until a powder is formed. Add the remaining ingredients and continue to blend, stopping the blender and scraping the sides every few minutes.

2. The process takes a while, around 15 minutes if you are not using a high-speed blender or around 10 if you do have one. You'll think that it's not turning into almond butter, but it does, and when it does, you'll be pleasantly surprised.

3. Store in a sealed jar in the fridge.

Note: Spread this butter on apple slices for a delicious snack.

Smashed Avocado on Toast

This is a filling yet light breakfast. The avocado spread is delicious and a great way to start the day, since it's loaded with healthy fats and plenty of fiber.

To have ease with meal prepping for the week, follow the recipe as written. Alternatively, toast your bread and add the smashed avocado (and optional egg) the morning of, for freshness.

Ingredients
1 large avocado
Juice of 1 lime
Pinch of red pepper flakes
4 thin slices paleo bread
Salt and pepper, to taste
2 eggs (optional)

Directions
1. In a bowl, add the flesh of the avocado, lime juice, and pinch of red pepper flakes. Mash well using a fork.
2. Toast four slices bread (two slices per serving), then spread the avocado mixture on top, dividing between your two servings. Sprinkle with salt and pepper.
3. If you're serving it with an egg for extra protein, cook the egg the way you like it. For a fried egg: add a teaspoon of olive oil to a skillet on high heat. Crack the egg into the pan. Cook for 3 minutes or until the edges begin to crisp. Season with salt and pepper.

Zoats

Zoats are a combination of zucchini and oats. I know that sounds a little weird, but I promise you will love it once you realize how good it tastes and how good it is for you. Play around with different toppings (such as berries or other fruits, or nuts), and use stevia instead of honey for a sugar-free alternative.

Ingredients
1 cup finely grated zucchini
½ cup uncooked oats
½ cup water
4 egg whites
2 to 3 teaspoons honey or 1 teaspoon stevia
2 tablespoons Maple Cinnamon Almond Butter (page 191)
½ teaspoon vanilla extract
2 teaspoons cinnamon (optional)
2 teaspoons maca powder (optional)
2 teaspoons cacao nibs (optional)

Directions

1. In a small saucepan, combine zucchini, oats, water, and egg whites. Cook, stirring constantly, on medium heat for 5 minutes.

2. Add honey or stevia, almond butter, maca powder and vanilla, stirring to combine.

3. Transfer to a bowl and top with cinnamon, maca powder, and/or cacao nibs. Cool, divide into two containers, and refrigerate.

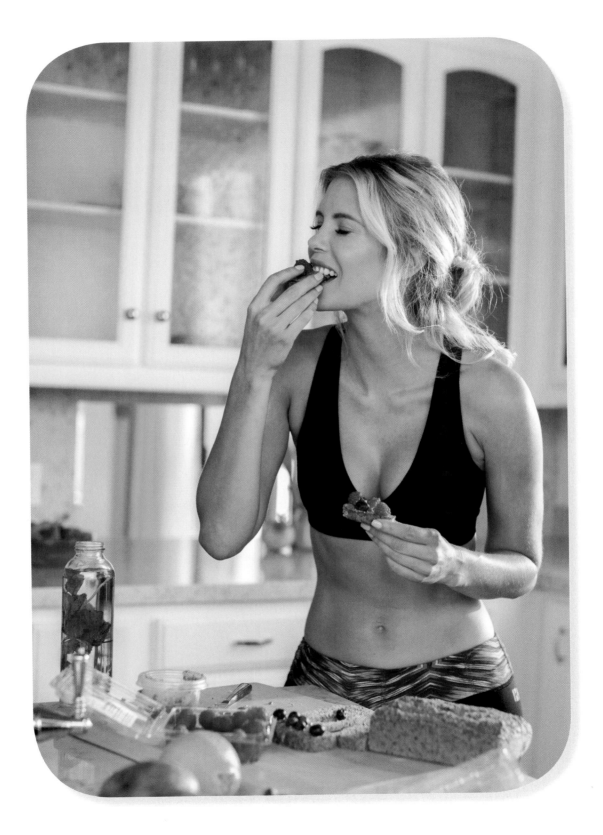

Maple Cinnamon Toast with Berries

Makes 1 serving

There is something so incredibly satisfying about toasted bread and any type of nut butter. Add cinnamon and berries (my favorites are sliced strawberries, mashed blueberries, and raspberries) and you have a winning breakfast that will leave your kitchen smelling incredible!

Ingredients

2 thicker or 3 thinner slices paleo bread
2 tablespoons Maple Cinnamon Almond Butter (page 191)
Cinnamon (optional)
½ cup berries

Directions

1. Toast the bread until lightly browned.
2. Spread the almond butter on top. Sprinkle on an additional pinch of cinnamon if desired. Top with berries.

Power Bowl

I call this dish Power Bowl because it is a powerful meal! It's hearty, satisfying, and will leave you feeling energized all day long. It's a complete meal, meaning that is has a good ratio of carbs to protein to fat, and is filled with vitamins. This is a great breakfast alternative when I'm tired of smoothies or sweeter breakfasts.

Ingredients
4 teaspoons olive oil
2 cups kale
1 cup cooked buckwheat groats
Dash of liquid aminos
½ tablespoon turmeric powder
1 teaspoon cayenne
2 eggs
6 cherry tomatoes, cut in half
Salt and pepper, to taste
Handful basil, chopped

Directions
1. Heat 2 teaspoons oil in a skillet on medium heat. Add the kale and sauté. Once it's almost cooked, add the buckwheat groats, liquid aminos, turmeric, and cayenne and mix well. Transfer to a bowl.
2. In the same pan, add another 2 teaspoons of olive oil. Beat the eggs and pour into the pan, mixing to scramble. Add the cherry tomatoes and cook lightly. Add salt and pepper to taste. Pour the cooked egg mixture onto the buckwheat groats and kale. Top with chopped basil.
3. Divide between 2 containers and refrigerate. To reheat, lightly sauté the mixture in a pan, or microwave for 60 seconds.

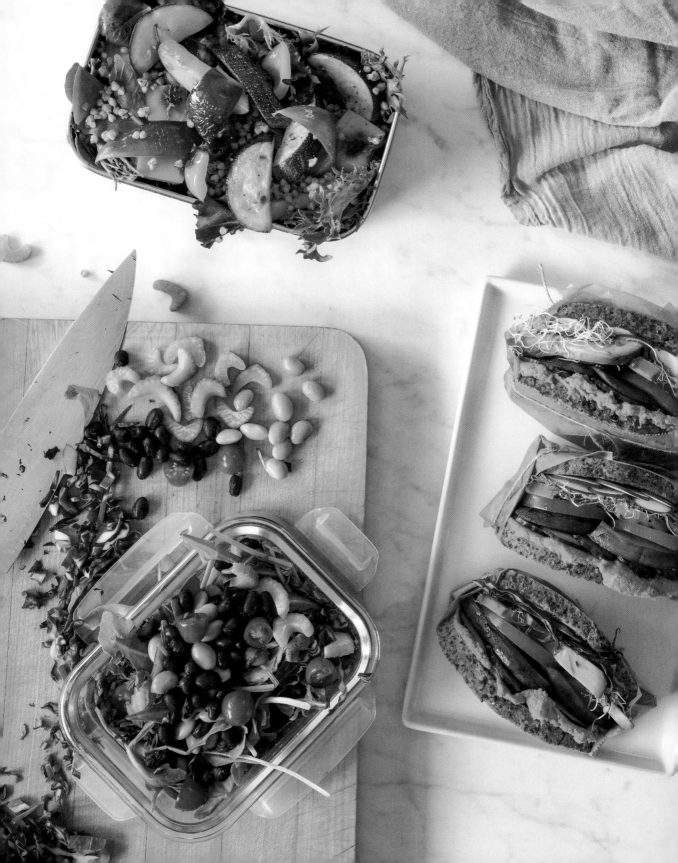

Lunches

Salad with Edamame and Black Beans

Makes 3 servings for the week

Simple and quick is best when it comes to meal prep—which is why I'm in love with this salad.

Ingredients
6 cups arugula or mixed greens
¾ cup cooked edamame
¾ cup black beans
¾ cup red cabbage, shredded
6 stalks celery, sliced
3 tablespoons black olives, chopped (not pictured)
6 cherry tomatoes, sliced (optional)
Salad dressing of choice—3 to 6 tablespoons (pages 251–253)

Directions
1. Add your arugula or mixed greens into three separate containers. Layer the remaining ingredients among each of them in equal portions.
2. Seal and place in fridge.
3. Serve with the salad dressing of your choice.

Paleo Sandwich with Hummus

Makes 2 servings for the week

Did I mention how much I love this bread? Wait until you try it with hummus and veggies as a sandwich. This is a super-versatile recipe too. You can add thinly sliced raw beets, shredded cabbage dressed with balsamic vinegar, and other colorful vegetables to give this sandwich a pop.

Ingredients
½ tablespoon olive oil
4 to 6 slices portobello mushroom
Salt and pepper, to taste
2 tablespoons Roasted Red Pepper Hummus (page 238)
4 slices paleo bread, toasted if desired
6 slices cucumber
1 tomato, sliced
Small handful alfalfa sprouts
½ avocado, sliced

Directions
1. Heat a pan on medium heat and add ½ tablespoon olive oil. Add mushroom slices and cook for 3 to 4 minutes, or until tender. Season with salt and pepper if desired.
2. Spread the hummus on one slice of bread.
3. Layer the mushroom slices, cucumber, tomato, alfalfa sprouts, and avocado on top of the hummus as well as any other vegetables. Place other slice of bread on top, and while pressing down, cut diagonally.

Tri-Colored Salad

Makes 2 servings for the week

As I've mentioned, salads are one of my favorite staples in meal prepping as well as a healthy diet because they are so easy to make and incredibly versatile. For the tri-colored salad, it's less important to follow the recipe exactly as written; rather, I'd like you to have three colors in your salad. If you'd like to add roasted vegetables, feel free—just make sure that you have three pops of color. If you'd like to use corn instead of tomatoes or garbanzo beans instead of black beans, feel free. Great additions include crumbled tempeh, leftover Miso-Glazed Salmon or Tempeh, pan-fried tofu, shredded chicken, or canned tuna.

Ingredients
4 handfuls spinach or arugula
15-ounce can black beans, drained and rinsed
½ cup cooked edamame
10 cherry tomatoes, chopped
3 red cabbage leaves, shredded
4 celery stalks, diced
Handful of cilantro, chopped
Salad dressing of choice—1 to 2 tablespoons (pages 251–253)

Directions
1. Divide the arugula among four different containers. On top of the arugula layer black beans, edamame, cherry tomatoes, cabbage, celery, and cilantro.
2. Top with dressing.

MEAL PREP YOUR WAY TO WEIGHT LOSS

200

Dinners

Zucchini Noodles with Hemp Pesto

Makes 2 servings for the week

Zucchini noodles, or "zoodles," are a fun meal to make, especially if you have kids (and I have found many hubbies enjoy them too). Zoodles are a low-carb alternative to noodles—and they're loaded with fiber, iron, and tons of flavor. This dish is one of my go-to dinners if I'm eating alone, or cooking for friends. If you'd like a slightly cheesier flavor, add a dusting of nutritional yeast flakes on top just before serving.

Ingredients
1 small package basil, chopped
1 cup spinach, chopped
¼ cup hemp seeds
2 garlic cloves, chopped
2 tablespoons nutritional yeast flakes
2 teaspoons cayenne
3 tablespoons olive oil + 1 teaspoon
4 zucchinis
5 slices tempeh, crumbled
1 tablespoon liquid aminos
1 handful cherry tomatoes, sliced

Directions

1. In a food processor or blender, combine basil, spinach, hemp seeds, garlic, nutritional yeast flakes, cayenne, and olive oil. Process until smooth, adding a little more olive oil if needed. Add salt and pepper if desired.

2. Using a spiralizer, spiralize all 4 zucchinis; add the pesto to the zucchini noodles and mix well with your hands. Divide between two separate containers.

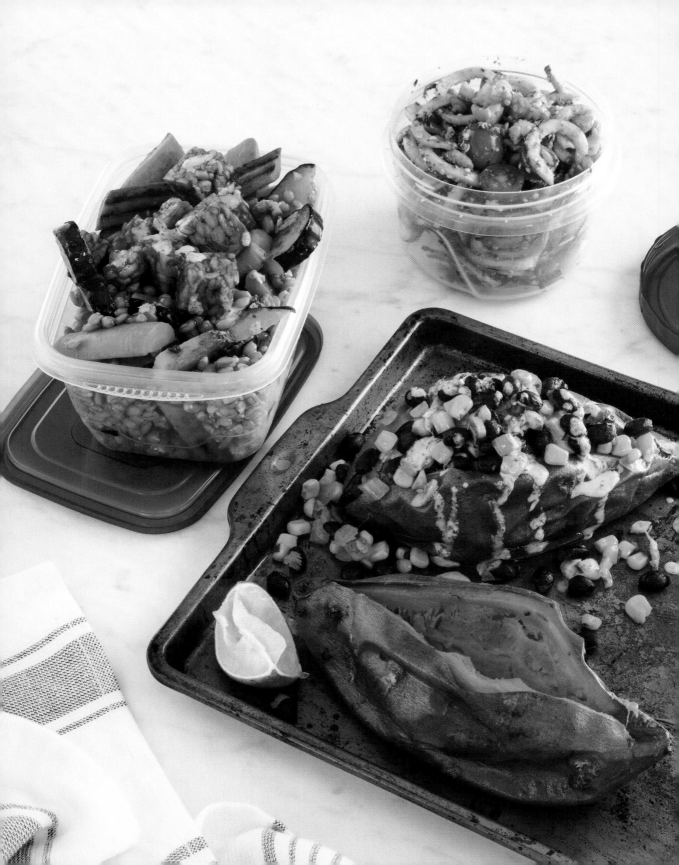

3. Heat 1 teaspoon olive oil in a pan over medium heat. Add the crumbled tempeh and 1 tablespoon liquid aminos and sauté lightly.

4. Divide the noodles, pesto, tempeh crumbles, and cherry tomatoes between two containers.

Loaded Mexican Baked Sweet Potato

Makes 2 servings for the week

Sweet potatoes have been known to get a bad rap because they are a carb. But the truth is, they won't spike your blood sugar like white potatoes do. (I'm not bashing white potatoes either; they're a natural carb that fit perfectly into a plant-based diet.) Sweet potatoes add color, natural sweetness, and a wide range of vitamins to your diet too. Served with the other vegetables in this meal, they won't leave you feeling weighed down like other baked potato recipes—and you'll be delighted by the taste.

Ingredients

2 sweet potatoes
1 tablespoon olive
2 garlic cloves, chopped
2 tablespoons finely chopped onion
½ cup black beans
½ cup corn
Pinch paprika
Salt and pepper, to taste
Juice of 2 limes
1 handful cilantro, finely chopped
Salad dressing of choice (optional)—1 to 2 tablespoons

Directions

1. Preheat the oven to 400 degrees. Slice each potato vertically, making sure you do not fully cut it into two pieces. Place on a baking dish and bake for 45 minutes or until the skin begins to get crispy and the inside is tender. Cool slightly.

2. In a small skillet, heat oil on medium-high heat. Sauté the garlic and onion until translucent.

3. Add the black beans, corn, and paprika and heat through. Season with salt and pepper.

4. Add half the lime juice to the black bean mixture, stirring to combine.

5. Top the potato halves with the black bean mixture. Top with chopped cilantro and drizzle with the remaining lime juice, and dressing of choice.

Roasted Vegetables with Spelt

I've changed this dish up a bit by adding spelt, a nutrient-rich and nutty-flavored whole grain. Here I used acorn squash, zucchini, and carrot, but you can use whatever vegetables you like. Remember to go for three colors in each meal.

Ingredients
1 cup roasted vegetables
6 2cm-sized slices tempeh, cubed
1 tablespoon olive oil
½ cup corn, drained and rinsed
1 tablespoon liquid aminos
1 cup cooked spelt
6 sprigs cilantro, chopped
Salad dressing of choice—1 to 2 tablespoons (pages 251–253)

Directions
1. Select the vegetables you'd like to roast, and cook according to roasting directions on page 39.

2. While the vegetables are roasting, cube or roughly chop the tempeh (or tofu), then add to a pan with 1 tablespoon olive oil over medium-high heat. After a minute shake the pan so the tempeh doesn't burn. Keep doing this until all sides are browned, around 5 minutes. Add corn to the

pan, along with the liquid aminos, and cook for 1 to 2 minutes until tempeh and corn are covered. Remove and cool.

3. Add the roasted veggies to a bowl with spelt, tempeh, and cilantro.

4. Toss with salad dressing of your choice (see pages 251–253)—1 to 2 tablespoons.

Sensational Stir-Fry

(See page 148)

Sensational Stir-Fry Sauce

(See page 148)

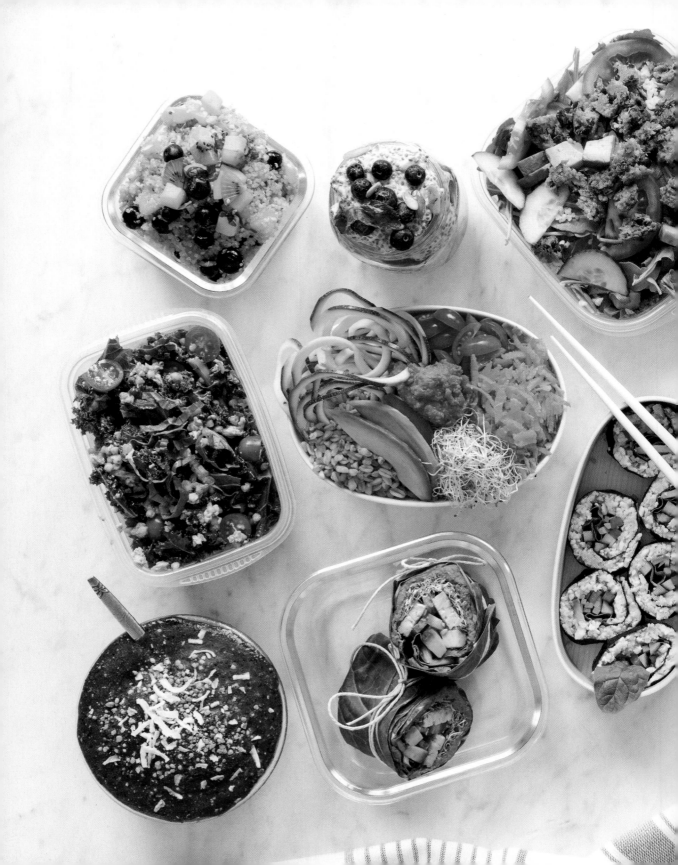

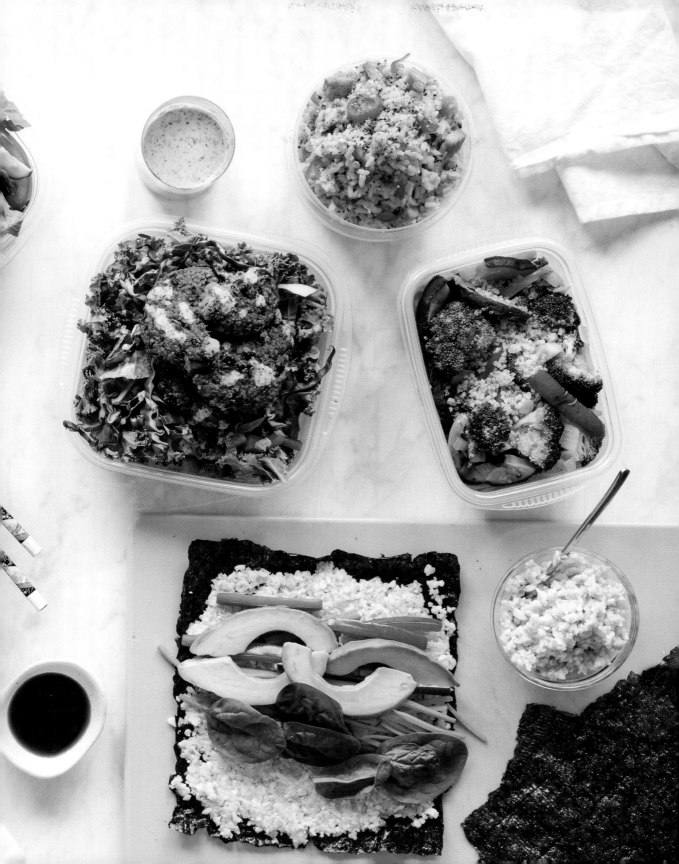

CHAPTER 14

Week Four—Detoxing

One of the most common questions I get is, "How can I lose weight fast?" We are living at a time when everything is so fast-paced, and we seem to demand everything *now*.

I answer that question in two ways. One is to do a detox, as outlined in my first book, *The 5-Day Real Food Detox*. It's healthy, nutritious, and satisfying; plus, you can lose up to a pound a day.

The other is to do a modified detox, which is week four of this plan. During this week, you'll be eating foods that are natural detoxifiers which help restore balance to your system. Don't worry—you won't be skimping on any food or starving yourself. Rather, you'll continue eating lots of real foods, all designed to cleanse your body. Please remember, though, that it takes time to see results that last, and quick fixes do not work for long-term success.

This part of the plan will help you break a plateau, which often occurs at the four-week mark in many weight-loss plans. And it can help you lose those last five stubborn pounds if that's what you need to do.

WEEK FOUR MEAL PLAN

	Monday	Tuesday	Wednesday	Thursday	Friday	Saturday	Sunday
Breakfast	Blueberry Ginger Smoothie Bowl	Blueberry Ginger Smoothie Bowl	Overnight Oats	Overnight Oats	Quinoa Lime Fruit Salad	Quinoa Lime Fruit Salad	Power Bowl
Lunch	Collard Wraps	Collard Wraps	Veggie Burger Inside Out	Veggie Burger Inside Out	Veggie Burger Inside Out	Rainbow Buddha Bowl	Rainbow Buddha Bowl
Dinner	Quinoa Black Bean Burgers	Quinoa Black Bean Burgers	Quinoa Black Bean Burgers	Cheesy Broccoli Rice	Cheesy Broccoli Rice	Sushi Rolls	Sensational Stir-Fry

Snacks: Choose two from Chapter 15

Grocery List for Week Four

Vegetables

Alfalfa sprouts, 1 small package

Arugula, 16-ounce package

Avocados, 5

Basil, 1 small package

Beet, 1

Bell peppers, red – 3

Bell pepper, any color – 1

Broccoli, 1 small head

Carrots, 5 large

Cauliflower, 1 head

Cherry tomatoes, 1 package

Cilantro, 1 bunch

Collard greens, enough for 2
large leaves

Cucumber, 2

Garlic, 1 bulb

Ginger root

Mint, 1 small package

Onions, 1 small

Spinach, 16-ounce package

Tomatoes, 4

Zucchini, 1

Fruits

Bananas, 2

Blueberries, fresh, 1 pint

Blueberries, frozen,
unsweetened, 12-ounce bag

Lemons, 3

Limes, 3

Mango, 1

Strawberries, 1 pint

Grains

Buckwheat groats, 16-ounce
package

Bulgur wheat, 24-ounce
package

Farro, 16-ounce package

Quinoa, 16-ounce package (or
brown rice, 16-ounce package)

Additional

Almond milk, 1 carton (or make
your own)

Black beans, 3 cans (15 ounces
each)

Edamame, shelled, frozen,
14-ounce package

Greek yogurt, plain, 6-ounce
carton

Nori seaweed wraps, 1 package

Tempeh, 6 slices

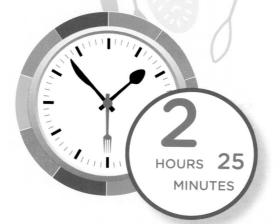

2 HOURS 25 MINUTES

Overview:
Meal Prep Timing—Week Four

5 minutes: Prepare area

10 minutes: Prep your grains

10 minutes: Prep the Blueberry Ginger Smoothie Bowl

5 minutes: Prep the Overnight Oats

10 minutes: Prep the Quinoa Lime Fruit Salad

15 minutes: Prep the Quinoa Power Bowl

10 minutes: Prep the Collard Wraps

10 minutes: Prep the Veggie Burger Inside Out

10 minutes: Prep the Rainbow Buddha Bowl

20 minutes: Prep the Quinoa Black Bean Burgers

15 minutes: Prep the Cheesy Broccoli Rice

10 minutes: Prep the Sushi Rolls

15 minutes: Prep the Sensational Stir-Fry

2 hours 25 minutes: total time*

*With optional snacks: Add 10 to 45 minutes to the total time

Meal Prep for Week Four

1. Several recipes this week call for cooked grains, and this part of prepping takes some ahead-of-time work. Cook enough quinoa to yield 5¼ cups (for the Quinoa Lime Fruit Salad, Quinoa Black Bean Burger, Cheesy Broccoli Rice, Sushi Rolls, and Sensational Stir-Fry); enough bulgur wheat for 2 cups (for the Veggie Burger Inside Out and Power Bowl); and enough farro to yield 1 cup (for the Rainbow Buddha Bowl). Prepare 1 cup of cooked brown rice if you're using it in the Cheesy Broccoli Rice instead of quinoa. Follow package directions or see instructions on page 96. You'll also need to have 1 cup of almond milk on hand.

2. Clear your area to make sure you have plenty of room for prepping. Gather together all your gadgets, cutlery, utensils, cookware, and containers.

3. Prep your breakfasts.

   - For the Blueberry Ginger Smoothie Bowl: You'll be prepping two servings.

     - Review the recipe.

     - Add all ingredients into a blender with ice and water, blending until smooth. Add smoothie into two mason jars or small containers and seal tight. Place in fridge.

   - For the Overnight Oats: You'll be prepping two servings.

     - Review the recipe.

     - Follow all the steps.

     - Divide the mixture into two bowls. Cover and refrigerate.

   - For the Quinoa Lime Salad: You'll be prepping two servings.

     - Review the recipe.

     - Chop the mango and herbs.

- Prepare the dressing.
- Combine the quinoa, berries, mango, and hemp seeds. Drizzle with dressing.
- Divide the mixture into two bowls. Cover and refrigerate.

- For the Quinoa Power Bowl: You'll be prepping one serving.
  - Review the recipe.
  - Complete steps 1 and 2. Reserve the avocado and basil until you are ready to serve the dish.
  - Divide into two containers. Seal well and refrigerate.

4. Prep your lunches.

- For the Collard Wraps: you'll be prepping two servings.
  - Review the recipe.
  - Shred the carrots, slice the tomatoes, and slice the tempeh.
  - Follow steps 1 to 3.
  - Cover Collard Wraps in plastic wrap and refrigerate until ready to serve.

- For the Veggie Burger Inside Out: You'll be prepping three servings.
  - Review the recipe.
  - Dice the cucumber and slice the avocado.
  - Cook your bulgur wheat by bringing 2 cups water to a boil. Remove from stove, and stir in 1 cup bulgur wheat. Cover and let stand for 20 minutes. Drain off any excess liquid; fluff with a fork, then transfer to another dish to cool.
  - Divide all ingredients into three separate containers, seal and refrigerate.

- For the Rainbow Buddha Bowl: You'll be prepping two servings.
  - Review the recipe.
  - Spiralize the zucchini, shred the 2 large carrots, and slice the 2 large tomatoes.
  - Divide the ingredients, including the farro, between two bowls. Seal and refrigerate.
  - When ready to serve, drizzle your Buddha bowl with your favorite salad dressing.

5. Prep your dinners.

  - For the Quinoa Black Bean Burgers: You'll be prepping three servings.
    - Review the recipe.
    - Create the "egg" chia if not using eggs.
    - Follow steps 2 through 8.
    - Let burgers cool. Place in containers and refrigerate.
    - When ready to serve, reheat in the microwave for 2 to 3 minutes per serving.
    - Serve with Cilantro Tahini Dressing (see page 252) and a side of mixed greens and ¼ avocado, sliced or drizzle salad with your favorite dressing.

  - For the Cheesy Broccoli Rice: You'll be prepping two servings.
    - Review the recipe.
    - Steam the broccoli. Halve the cherry tomatoes.
    - Slice the tempeh into 6 slices. Sauté the tempeh as directed.
    - Add the rice to the broccoli and mix in the nutritional yeast flakes.

- Divide the mixture and transfer to two separate bowls. Top each with cherry tomatoes. Seal and refrigerate.

- For the Sushi Rolls: You'll be prepping one serving.
  - Review the recipe.
  - Make the cauliflower rice, as directed.
  - Slice the cucumber and carrot lengthwise. Cut the red bell pepper into 4 strips.
  - Layer the seaweed wraps with cauliflower rice and quinoa. Place the rest of the ingredients over the rice and quinoa. Wrap as directed.

- For the Sensational Stir-Fry, you'll be prepping one serving.
  - Review the recipe.
  - Chop all vegetables: broccoli, bell pepper, onion, and portobello mushroom. Cook the vegetables.
  - Cook the quinoa.
  - Prepare the sauce.
  - Mix together the veggies, quinoa, and sauce. Place in a container. Seal well and refrigerate.
  - Reheat and garnish with chopped basil.

6. Clean up. If you clean up as you go, you'll save time in the end.

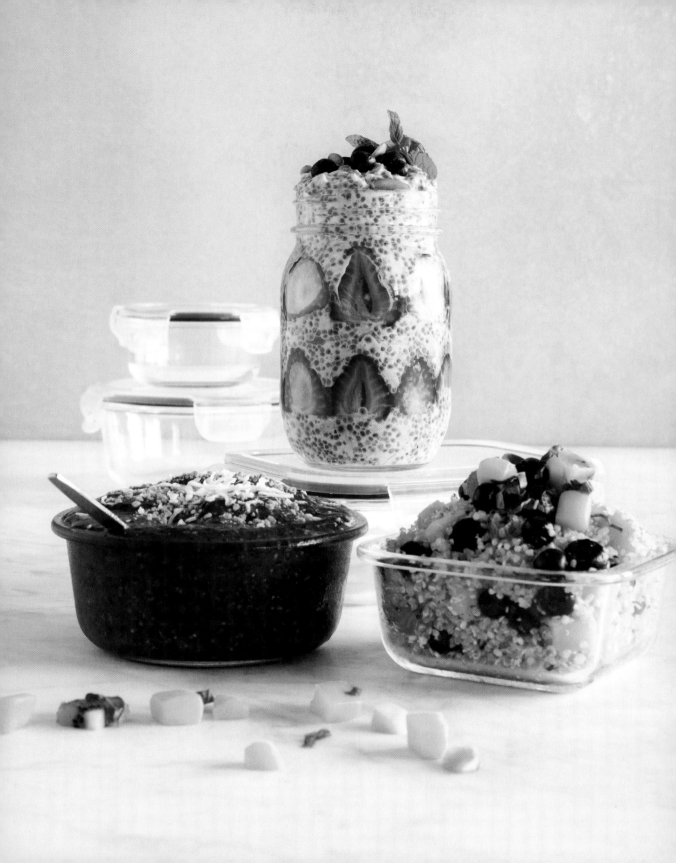

Breakfasts

Blueberry Ginger Smoothie Bowl

Makes 2 servings for the week

Smoothie bowls fill you up, cool you down, and contain plenty of water and fruits to keep you hydrated. If that's not enough of a reason to blend up this baby, the Blueberry Ginger Smoothie Bowl is also packed with antioxidants to support immune health and help neutralize free radicals in the body. You can top these with whatever garnishes you like; I recommend cacao nibs, bee pollen, coconut flakes, and goji berries.

Ingredients
Two large handfuls spinach
2 bananas
2 cups frozen blueberries
½-inch fresh ginger, peeled
2 teaspoons turmeric powder*
2 tablespoons chia seeds
½ cup uncooked oats
1 tablespoon spirulina

Directions
1. Place all ingredients into a blender, along with 1.5 cups water and a handful of ice. Blend until smooth. If you'd like it a thinner consistency, add more water.
2. Pour into mason jars and seal, placing them into the fridge. When serving, garnish with your choice of toppings.

*I recommend ½-inch fresh turmeric root for this recipe; however, it can be costly and hard to find. If available to you, swap powder for fresh turmeric.

Overnight Oats

Overnight oats have been popular for quite some time, and for good reason: they're the perfect breakfast for busy people! Mix your ingredients, throw the concoction in the fridge, then either grab and go the next morning or layer it up with different fruits and other tasty toppings before heading out the door. Try more cinnamon, pumpkin seeds, a sliced kiwi, or a tablespoon of Maple Cinnamon Almond Butter (page 191). The longer you let overnight oats sit, the thicker the mixture will get.

Ingredients
½ cup rolled oats
2 tablespoons chia seeds
½ teaspoon cinnamon
1 cup almond milk
½ teaspoon vanilla extract
2 cups blueberries

Directions
1. Mix together oats, chia seeds, cinnamon, almond milk, and vanilla extract in a large bowl and stir. Add blueberries and stir again. Divide mixture into two mason jars. Cover each with plastic wrap and place in the fridge.
2. The next morning, stir and eat.

Quinoa Lime Fruit Salad

Makes 2 servings for the week

You've used quinoa only in savory meals, such as salads and stir-fries, right? Well, it's time to change it up and eat it for breakfast! This is going to change your perception on this delicious grain. Note that in the photo of the Quinoa Lime Fruit Salad (page 217) I used kiwi instead of strawberries. You can switch up the fruit you use—instead of strawberries try diced apple, cherries, or whatever else you have on hand.

Ingredients
½ cup cooked quinoa
½ cup blueberries
½ cup strawberries
½ cup diced mango
2 tablespoons hemp seeds
Juice of 2 limes
2 teaspoons honey
2 tablespoons chopped basil
2 tablespoons chopped mint
2 teaspoons bee pollen (optional)

Directions
1. In a bowl, combine quinoa, fruit, and hemp seeds.
2. In a separate bowl, mix together lime juice and honey, along with a pinch of the basil and mint, whisking until the honey has combined well.
3. Drizzle the lime and honey mixture over the quinoa and fruit, topping with remaining chopped basil and mint. Add bee pollen if using.
4. Divide the mixture into two bowls. Cover and refrigerate.

Power Bowl

Makes 1 serving for the week (See page 196.)

I wanted to include a recipe from week 3 that is a savory and satiating breakfast. You'll be using bulgur wheat, instead of millet to switch it up. As this is only one serving, you'll use ½ cup; however, feel free to use less if desired. And remember, you can swap out the vegetables and replace the egg with vegan protein!

Lunches

Collard Wraps

Makes 2 servings for the week

Collard wraps are a great alternative to a sandwich or a burrito, and they are delicious no matter what filling you use. If you don't care for tempeh, for example, fill the wraps with "taco meat": 1 cup walnuts, 2 tablespoons liquid aminos, 1 tablespoon miso, and a dash of turmeric. Add in dried herbs such as basil, rosemary, and so forth. Combine these ingredients in a food processor until a meat-like consistency is achieved. Or try adding roasted portobello mushrooms. The varieties are endless, and you'll soon find that these are easy to make and a great on-the-go meal.

Ingredients
2 large collard leaves
4 tablespoons Creamy Beet Dip (page 239)
2 large carrots, shredded
4 slices miso-glazed tempeh (recipe page 176)
2 small tomatoes, sliced
Small handful alfalfa sprouts
6 springs cilantro
½ avocado, sliced

Directions
1. Place the collard leaf flat on a cutting board and cut vertically on both sides of the tough stem to remove it, leaving you with two smaller leaves. Place one leaf about halfway over a second leaf to create a single larger wrap. Repeat with the remaining leaves.
2. Spread each wrap with half the beet dip. Divide the remaining ingredients between the two wraps.

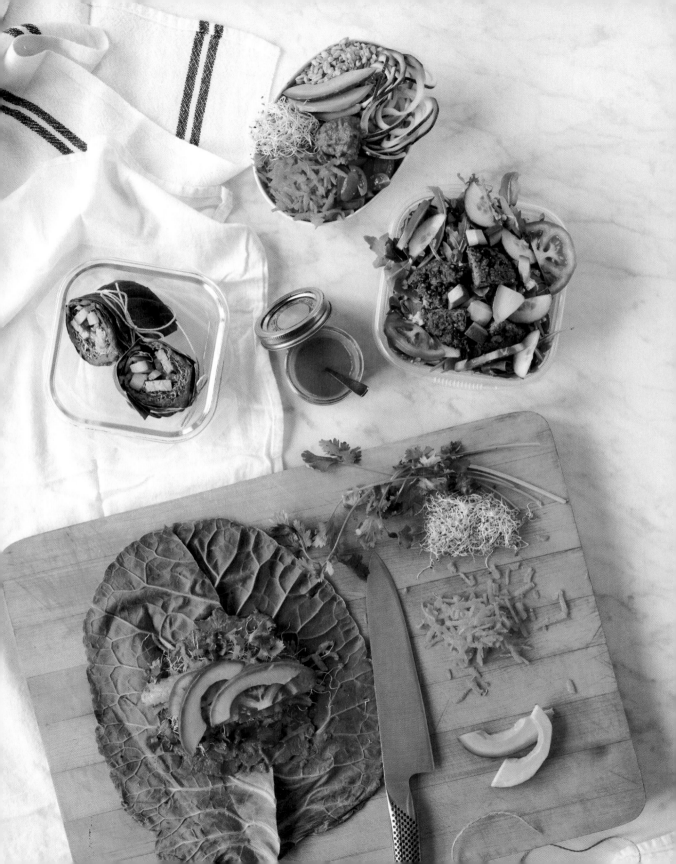

3. Roll up the leaves as you would a burrito: start rolling from one long side and fold the shorter ends over as you go, making sure nothing spills out. Cut each wrap in half. Use a toothpick to hold the wraps together if desired.

Veggie Burger Inside Out

Makes 3 servings for the week

Here's a beautifully simple meal that tastes wonderful and is good for your digestive system—a must when you're detoxing. The lemon juice and olive oil dressing adds an extra burst of freshness and is one of my favorite ways to dress a salad, though you can try any of the dressings in this book (pages 251–253). You can also swap out the bulgur for brown rice, quinoa, or any super grain.

Ingredients
1½ cups cooked bulgur wheat
3 cups arugula
6-inch piece cucumber, chopped
2 avocados, sliced
3 Quinoa Black Bean Burgers (page 226)
3 tablespoons olive oil
Juice of 1 to 2 lemons
Salt and pepper, to taste

Directions
1. Combine the cooked bulgur, arugula, cucumber, and avocado into three containers.
2. Break up the Quinoa Black Bean burger patties into bite-sized pieces and add one per container. Seal and refrigerate.
3. When ready to serve, drizzle with the oil and lemon juice, season with salt and pepper, and toss.

Rainbow Buddha Bowl

Makes 2 servings for the week

Buddha Bowls truly are one of my favorite meals because they are so incredibly versatile and perfect for any meal of the day. Feel free to add any super herbs, such as cilantro, basil, or parsley. Swap out the large tomatoes for 6 sliced cherry tomatoes if desired, which are pictured.

Ingredients
1 zucchini, spiralized
2 large tomatoes, sliced
1 cup cooked farro
3 tablespoons Creamy Beet Dip (page 239)
2 large carrots, shredded
½ avocado, sliced
Small handful alfalfa sprouts
Salad dressing of choice (pages 251–253)

Directions

1. Divide the spiralized zucchini between two bowls, keeping it to one side. Next, slice the tomatoes and put one in each bowl, next to the zucchini. Repeat this process with the farro, beet dip, carrots, avocado, and sprouts.

2. Prior to serving, top with your dressing of choice—1 to 2 tablespoons.

Dinners

Quinoa Black Bean Burgers

Makes 3 servings for the week (1 serving is 2 burgers)
plus 3 to be saved for the Veggie Burger Inside Out for lunch.

Usually I bake these burgers, as directed below, but you can also fry them in a skillet with a little olive oil on medium heat, five minutes on each side. They cook quickly and can sometimes burn if you're not watching. I've set off my smoke detector a few times—which is why I prefer baking them! The recipe makes enough for three days' worth, however you will have leftovers, which are perfect to freeze, then reheat or snack on, as well as add to other salads. In the photo, I served these with kale, purple cabbage, and red pepper; however, feel free to add any super vegetables you'd like, or roasted veggies, and serve with the dressing of your choice.

Ingredients
1 tablespoon olive oil, and some for greasing
3 cups cooked quinoa
1 small onion, finely chopped
2 garlic cloves, finely chopped
1 ½ small red peppers, seeded and finely chopped
3 cans (15 ounces each) black beans, drained and rinsed
1 ½ cups spinach, chopped
¾ teaspoon paprika
¾ teaspoon salt
¾ teaspoon pepper
½ teaspoon cayenne (optional)
½ teaspoon turmeric powder (optional)
3 eggs (or 3 chia "eggs"; see sidebar)
1 cup oat flour*

*To create oat flour, take 1 cup rolled oats and blitz in your blender, making sure it's fully dry before doing so. This is an incredibly cheap alternative to buying oat flour.

Directions

1. Preheat the oven to 375 degrees.
2. Cover a baking sheet with foil and grease the foil lightly with olive oil.
3. If the quinoa is not still warm, reheat it (add the quinoa to a pan with a dash of water or apple cider vinegar and heat through).
4. Sauté the onion and garlic in olive oil, followed by the red pepper.
5. Place the beans in a bowl and lightly mash.
6. Combine the beans, quinoa, spinach, and spices and mix well. Add the eggs and oat flour and mix well.
7. Place a palm-sized amount of this mixture in your hand and form into a patty. You should get about 9 patties.
8. Bake in the oven, 20 minutes on each side.
9. Remove from oven. Let cool. Place in containers and refrigerate. When ready to serve, reheat in the microwave for 2 to 3 minutes, or in the oven under the broiler for 1 to 2 minutes.

CHIA "EGGS"

Vegans or people with egg allergies can substitute chia "eggs" in the Quinoa Black Bean Burgers. To make the equivalent of 3 eggs, combine 3 tablespoons ground chia seeds with 9 tablespoons water in a small bowl. Mix and allow to sit for at least 15 minutes before using in the recipe.

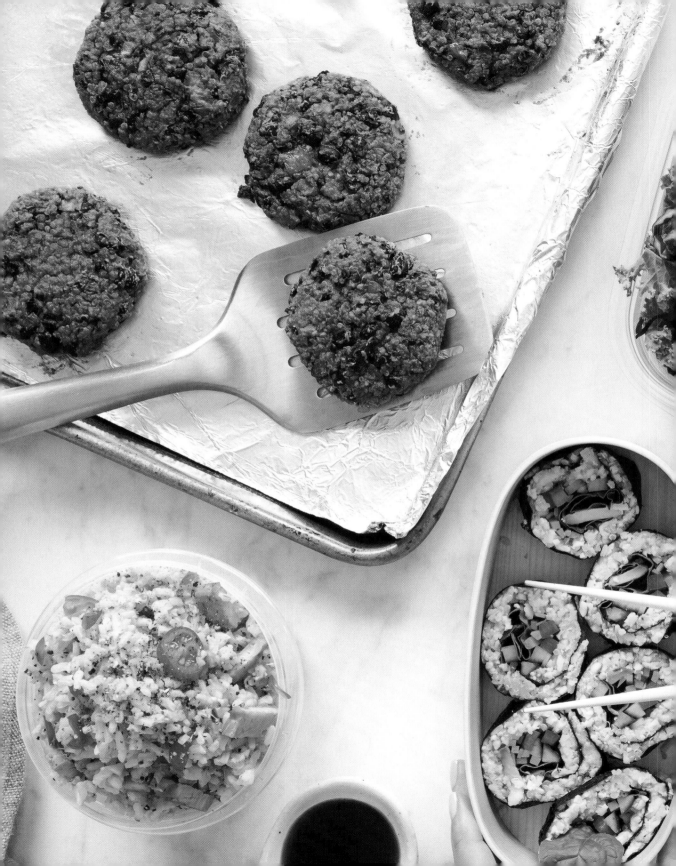

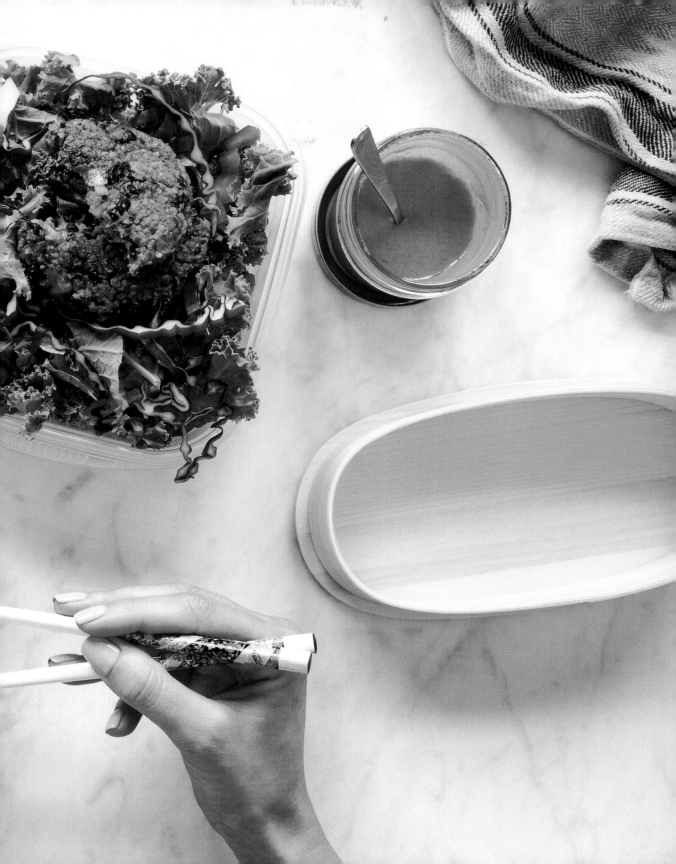

Cheesy Broccoli Rice

Makes 2 servings for the week

Dinner doesn't have to be complicated, which is why I love this recipe. It's quick, especially if you have the brown rice or quinoa already made, and it can be topped with any protein you'd like. I tend to go for tempeh or a lightly fried egg, but feel free to swap out the tempeh for whatever you like, or include more vegetables.

Ingredients
1 tablespoon olive oil
1 cup cooked brown rice or quinoa
1 cup steamed broccoli
4 tablespoons nutritional yeast flakes
Salt and pepper, to taste
2 handfuls cherry tomatoes, sliced
4 slices tempeh
1 tablespoon liquid aminos

Directions
1. Heat olive oil in a pan on medium-high. Add brown rice or quinoa and heat through.
2. Add the broccoli and nutritional yeast flakes (which is where the cheesy flavor comes from). Mix well. Season with salt and pepper. Transfer to two bowls and divide the cherry tomatoes between the bowls.
3. In the same pan, sauté the tempeh in the liquid aminos 2 minutes each side. Add to the rice and broccoli mixture.

Sushi Rolls

Here's a recipe from my *5-Day Real Food Detox* that has been a big hit. Dip the rolls in liquid aminos instead of soy sauce, and you've got yourself a tasty and much healthier alternative to restaurant sushi. I love to swap out ingredients here, so if you don't like a certain ingredient or want to add something else, feel free.

Ingredients
1 cup cauliflower rice (see sidebar, page 232)
½ cup cooked quinoa
2 nori seaweed wraps
¼ cucumber, sliced lengthwise into strips
1 large carrot, sliced lengthwise
10 strips red bell pepper
½ avocado
Small handful spinach

Directions
1. Mix the cauliflower rice and quinoa in a bowl.
2. Place the nori seaweed wrap shiny-side up. Using your fingers, spread ½ the cauliflower mixture evenly over the wrap from the bottom edge (the edge closest to you) up to about 1 inch from the top. Leave a 1-inch strip of the wrap at the top edge (the edge farthest from you) bare.
3. Place half of the remaining ingredients along the bottom edge of the nori sheet (the edge closest to you). Starting at the bottom edge, roll tightly. Cut the finished roll into 1-inch slices.
4. Repeat with the second nori sheet and the other half of the ingredients.
Note: As an option, add slices of purple cabbage and chopped cilantro leaves in addition to the ingredients listed above for extra color, texture, and taste in your sushi rolls.

HOW TO PREP CAULIFLOWER RICE

Chop the stem and leaves off ½ head cauliflower. Cut into chunks and process in a food processor or blender until the cauliflower is finely chopped and looks like rice. You can also do this by hand using a grater. Put the cauliflower into a pan and cook on medium heat for 5 minutes, stirring constantly, until soft. (Alternatively, place in a bowl and microwave for 3 minutes or until soft.) If you're using it for sushi, transfer the cauliflower to a cloth towel and wring out any excess moisture. The cauliflower rice can be stored in a covered container in the refrigerator.

Sensational Stir-Fry

(See page 148.)

Sensational Stir-Fry Sauce

(See page 148.)

CHAPTER 15
Prepping Snacks, Desserts, and More

Snacking and eating desserts have long gotten a bad rap; more often than not, they're viewed as little more than an opportunity to eat lots of calories, fat, sugar, and sodium. But snacks and desserts—as long as they're healthy—are an important part of a nutritious diet, and healthy lifestyle.

Snacking is a great weight control tool too. Studies show that nutritious snacking can tame hunger and prevent overeating at main meals. It can also play an important role in controlling cravings, especially if you plan to have a snack at predictable times, such as midmorning and midafternoon.

Need proof? A 2011 study published in the *Nutrition Journal* found that the inclusion of low-sugar, moderately high-protein snacks helped to reduce body weight and boost fat loss in type 2 diabetes patients. And a study published in the *British Journal of Nutrition* found that people who ate a high-protein, moderate-calorie snack (in this case, cheese) one hour before lunch automatically cut back their calories during subsequent meals on the same day. This means that smart snacking is a great way to rein in an out-of-control appetite.

If you make healthy choices, snacks and desserts can also make significant contributions to the nutritional quality of your diet. The key is to stick with mostly nutrient-dense foods such as fruits, vegetables, nuts, and seeds—all packed with vitamins, minerals, antioxidants, phytochemicals, and fiber.

PREP THESE SNACK SUGGESTIONS

Besides the recipes I've included in this chapter, here are some quick-and-easy-to-prep suggestions for healthy snacking:

- Nut butter on apple slices
- Chopped raw broccoli or cauliflower with one of my salad dressings for dipping
- Black bean salsa served with celery sticks, baby carrots, or sliced cucumbers
- Fresh fruit, washed and cut up, with a little Greek, soy, or coconut yogurt for dipping
- Hard-boiled egg with chopped raw veggies
- Raw veggie slices with hummus
- Mixtures of raw nuts, seeds, and dried fruit
- Vegetable and fruit smoothie with nut milk and vegan protein powder

As for my snacks, each one is simple to prep, package up, and take with you to school or work. You get to enjoy two snacks a day—if you wish. Keep in mind that snacks are optional but recommended.

I recommend choosing what snacks you'd like for the week, then portion them out with Ziploc baggies or containers.

If you opt to make any of my snacks, be sure to review the ingredients and add them to your weekly grocery list.

In this chapter, you'll also find my recipes for salad dressings. They're all natural and highly nutritious—none of the additives or preservatives commonly found in bottled dressings. Plus they're a cinch to prep and store. I like to divide my dressings into single-serving containers so that they're ready to go.

On this plan, you're allowed one dessert a week, and like the snacks, they're optional. I confess to having a sweet tooth, so I love having my desserts. But I know all too well what conventional desserts can do to your waistline and health. Thus I've spent years experimenting with dessert recipes that taste incredible but don't contain the high levels of sugar and fat of traditional desserts. I've learned how to maximize the natural sweetness in fruit, and I use super ingredients such as cacao nibs, coconut, and other delights to create delicious, nutrient-rich concoctions. The other great thing about these desserts is that, unlike the sugar-laden stuff, they will fill you up, even after a few small bites. That's because they're high in satisfying fiber and palate-pleasing natural ingredients.

A reminder: If you choose to enjoy your weekly dessert, be sure to review the ingredients and add them to your weekly grocery list.

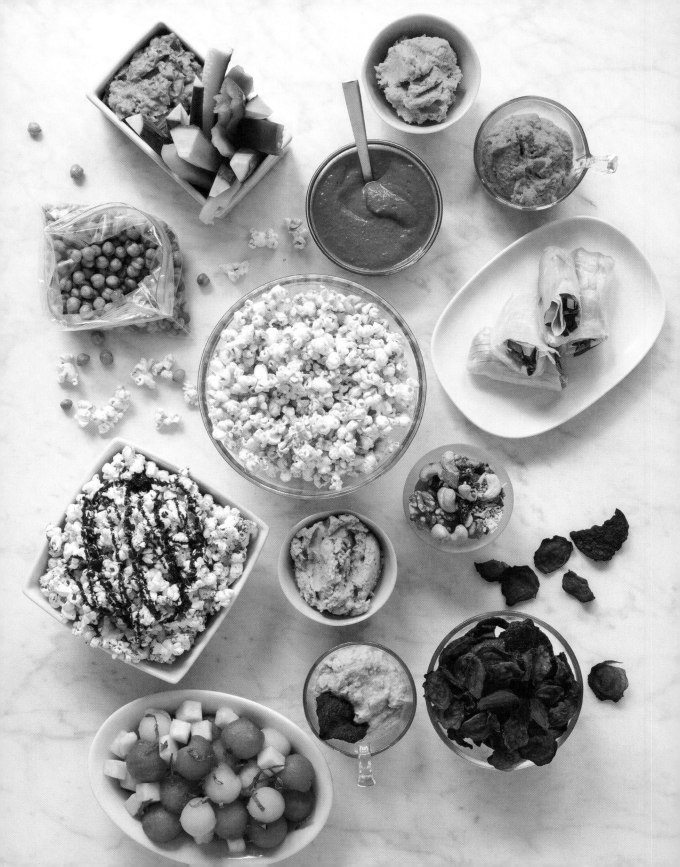

Super Snacks

The Best Hummus and Beet Chips

Makes 1 batch for the week (a single serving is ¼ cup)

This hummus recipe is beyond good! It tastes so much better than anything store-bought, and it's a cinch to make. Simplicity is key here.

The beet chips don't have any of the unhealthy calories of regular chips, but they taste just as good and give you that delicious crunch that normal chips do.

Ingredients
1 can (15 ounces) chickpeas, drained and rinsed
1 tablespoon tahini
Juice of 1 lemon
2 tablespoons olive oil
½ teaspoon turmeric
½ teaspoon salt
Pepper, to taste
2 large beets, peeled

Directions
1. In a blender, combine chickpeas, tahini, lemon juice, 1 tablespoon oil, ½ teaspoon turmeric, and ½ teaspoon salt. Blend until smooth. Taste and adjust salt and lemon juice as needed; season with pepper. Adjust the consistency with a little water or olive oil if needed.
2. Preheat the oven to 375 degrees.
3. Using a mandoline, slice beets on the thicker side, around the level 3 on the mandoline. Using a mandoline will help ensure that the beet slices are all the same thickness, which is important for even cooking.
4. Arrange the beet chips, not touching, on a paper towel. Cover with a

237

second paper towel and microwave for 45 seconds. Pat to remove excess water.

5. Place the beet chips in a single layer on a parchment-lined baking sheet. Drizzle with the remaining 1 tablespoon olive oil (you can also mix the beet slices and the oil in a bowl before spreading them on the baking sheet). Sprinkle with salt and pepper.

6. Bake for 15 to 20 minutes, checking them at 15 minutes to make sure they don't burn. Remove from oven and let cool. Serve with the hummus. To store, place the chips in an airtight container with a piece of paper towel to absorb excess moisture; the hummus should be refrigerated.

Roasted Red Pepper Hummus

Makes 1 batch for the week (a single serving is ¼ cup)

Ingredients
1 red bell pepper
1 can (15 ounces) chickpeas, drained and rinsed
1 tablespoon tahini
Juice of 1 lemon
1 tablespoon olive oil
½ teaspoon cayenne
Salt and pepper, to taste

Directions
1. Preheat broiler. Place red pepper on a lined baking sheet and broil until the skin begins to blister. Flip the pepper and continue broiling another few minutes, carefully watching, until the second side is blistered. Remove and allow to cool. Remove the stem and seeds and peel the skin off.

2. Place the cooled roasted pepper into a blender or food processor, add the remaining ingredients, season with salt and pepper, and blend until smooth. Adjust the consistency with a little water or olive oil if needed.

Creamy Beet Dip

Clean eating shouldn't be boring. It's all about playing with different flavors, textures, and colors to satisfy your eyes, mouth, and tummy—and this dip does it all. Note that it does use a little Greek yogurt, so if you're vegan, use the same quantity of soft tofu or soy yogurt in its place. For the Collard Wraps (page 222), I added ½ cup cooked chickpeas to the Creamy Beet Dip mixture and blended to make it thicker. Serve with chopped veggies, or use as a spread on sandwiches, instead of mayonnaise.

Ingredients
1 large beet
3 tablespoons Greek yogurt
½ teaspoon turmeric powder
½ teaspoon cayenne
Juice of ½ lemon

Directions
1. Peel the beet, chop it, and add the pieces to a pot of boiling water. Cook until a fork goes through them easily and they are very soft. Drain and allow to cool. (Alternatively, roast the beet chunks.)
2. Place the cooked beets and all other ingredients in a food processor and process until smooth. Season with salt and pepper.
3. Place the mixture in a container. Seal well and refrigerate.

Lite Babaganoush

This Mediterranean-inspired dip is a delicious blend of healthy ingredients and is a cinch to make. It's usually served with pita bread, but raw veggies—carrot sticks, cucumber slices, or celery sticks—taste just as good and are infinitely more filling. Also try dipping with Beet Chips (page 237).

Ingredients
1 pound eggplant
2 garlic cloves
2 tablespoons tahini
½ teaspoon ground cumin
1 teaspoon salt
Juice of ½ lemon

Directions

1. Preheat the broiler. Place the eggplant on a baking sheet and prick deeply with a fork. Broil for 18 to 20 minutes, until the skin looks slightly charred.

2. Remove the eggplant and transfer it to a plate to cool. Put the garlic on the baking sheet and broil for 2 minutes until roasted and lightly browned. Remove and allow to cool.

3. Run eggplant under cool water and rub to remove the skin. Cut the eggplant into small pieces, then place in a dish towel and squeeze out excess moisture.

4. Combine the eggplant, garlic, and remaining ingredients in a blender or food processor and blend until smooth.

5. Place in a container and refrigerate until ready to serve.

Garlic and White Bean Dip

Makes 1 batch for the week (a single serving is ¼ cup)

For a quick-prep dip, this one is a winner. It takes no more than 5 minutes to make and can be refrigerated for up to a week. Serve with raw carrot sticks, cucumber slices, and celery sticks.

Ingredients

1 can (15 ounces) butter beans, drained and rinsed
2 garlic cloves
Juice of ½ lemon
2 tablespoons olive oil
½ teaspoon oregano

Directions

1. Place all ingredients in a blender or food processor. Season with salt and pepper. Blend until smooth.
2. Transfer dip to a container and refrigerate until ready to serve.

Summer Spring Rolls

Makes 1 serving for the week

These are great when you find yourself craving an unhealthy wrap or burrito—they are light, filling, and won't leave you feeling heavy. The photo on page 236 shows a variety of ingredients you can add, so feel free to play around with different flavors and colors. When ready to snack, dip the rolls in liquid aminos or dressing of choice (pages 251–253).

Ingredients
2 rice paper wraps
2 large iceberg lettuce leaves
1 large carrot, julienned
1 inch cucumber, julienned
1 purple cabbage leaf, shredded
½ avocado, chopped
¼ red pepper, julienned
Small handful of cilantro, chopped

Directions
1. Heat a large pan of water to boiling. You only need about an inch of water, but it should be able to comfortably fit the entire rice paper inside without folding.
2. Place one rice paper wrap in the water, pulling it out after a few seconds (it should be soft).
3. Lay the rice wrap on a flat surface. Place one lettuce leaf in the center. Place half the vegetables in a line in the center. Sprinkle with half the cilantro.
4. Grab one side of the rice wrap and fold over the vegetables in the center. Fold the edges in and keep wrapping, making sure it's tight.
5. Repeat with the second rice wrap and the remaining ingredients.
6. Place the wraps in a container. Seal and refrigerate.

Melon Ball Fruit Salad

Makes 3 servings

I recommend purchasing a melon baller, as they are cheap and make food super fun to play with. You can buy them at Target, Amazon, or housewares stores. It takes an otherwise boring fruit salad and makes it very appealing. I haven't given specific amounts on the fruit, as you might buy a whole watermelon, pineapple, etc. However, I recommend using ½ of each fruit, with the option to buy precut pineapple, as you won't be using the melon baller for that.

Ingredients
Cantaloupe, watermelon, and pineapple
5 mint leaves, finely chopped

Directions
1. Use the baller on the cantaloupe and watermelon as you would an ice cream scoop (that's essentially what it is, but just a smaller version). Chop the pineapple. Place all the fruit in a bowl.
2. Mix the mint into the salad.
3. Either keep in one bowl and take out portions as needed, or divide into three containers. Cover the container with plastic wrap, then place the lid on top. This will last in the fridge for up to five days.

Homemade Guacamole

Makes 4 servings for the week

My mom taught me that simplicity is the key to creating amazing dishes. Thanks, Mom! It's all about taking food in its natural state and adding other simple ingredients to create fresh and delicious flavors. I suggest dipping cut-up raw veggies in this guacamole for a super-healthy, filling snack—prep the veggies in advance and portion them into baggies.

Ingredients
2 avocados
Juice of 1 lime
Salt and pepper, to taste
6 cilantro sprigs, finely chopped

Directions
1. Cut the avocados in half. Remove the pit and, using a spoon, scoop out all the flesh. Place in a bowl.
2. Add the lime juice to the avocado and season with salt and pepper. Mash the mixture with a fork. Mix in the chopped cilantro.
3. Place the mixture in a container and top with plastic wrap, pressing the wrap onto the surface of the guacamole in order to seal out excess air and prevent browning. Add the lid and refrigerate.

Crunchy Chickpeas

Here's a great snack to enjoy during the protein week of my plan or any week, for that matter! Chickpeas are loaded with protein and fiber, and cooked like this, they're better than peanuts or potato chips any day. You can pick any herb or spice you like—I'm a fan of za'atar, chili powder, curry powder, and smoked paprika—but I recommend you use only one spice per batch, for best flavor.

Ingredients
1 15-ounce can chickpeas, drained and rinsed
1 tablespoon olive oil
½ teaspoon salt
Pepper, to taste
2 teaspoons herb or spice of choice

Directions
1. Preheat the oven to 400 degrees.
2. Place the chickpeas between two kitchen towels and rub, to dry them as much as possible.
3. Place the chickpeas in a bowl. Add olive oil and salt and toss. Season with pepper to taste. Spread the chickpeas evenly on a baking sheet.
4. Bake for 20 to 30 minutes, shaking the pan after 10 minutes. The chickpeas will be golden brown when done.
5. Remove from the oven and toss with the herb or spice.

Prep tip: These are best eaten immediately after being baked, but you can store them in an airtight container to keep in your pantry. Then reheat them by placing them under the broiler for a few minutes. You can also toss a few onto salads or the Buddha Bowls throughout the week.

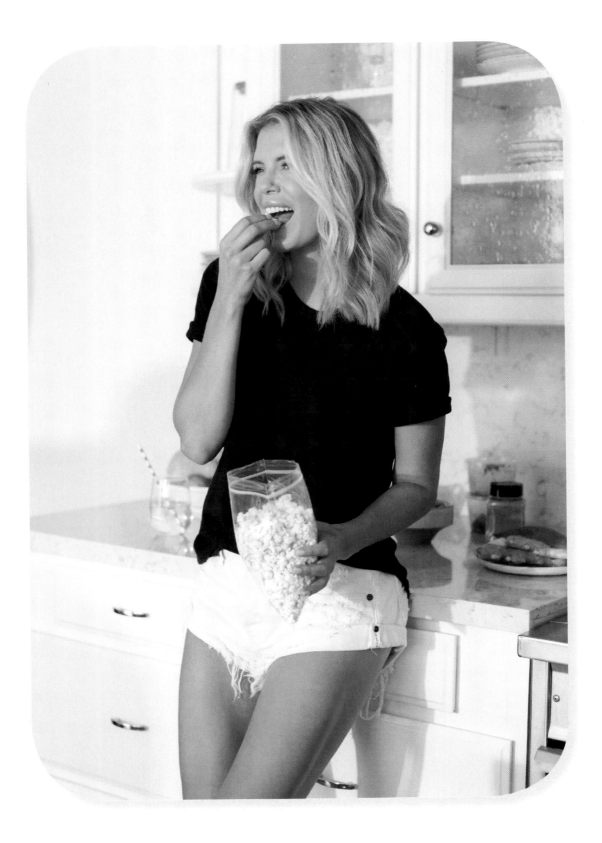

Cheesy Popcorn

Makes 1 serving

Craving popcorn? Look no further! This recipe is my go-to for snacking, movie-watching, and traveling.

Ingredients

2 tablespoons coconut oil
2 tablespoons popcorn kernels
1 tablespoon nutritional yeast flakes
Salt, to taste

Directions

1. Melt 1 tablespoon coconut oil in a large pot over medium-high heat. Add kernels and cover, shaking the pot occasionally, until you hear popping. Turn heat off once there is a long time between the sounds of popping.

2. Melt the second tablespoon of coconut oil in the microwave if it's not liquid, then drizzle over the popcorn. Sprinkle with the nutritional yeast flakes and season with salt. Mix with your hands.

Sweet 'n' Salty Popcorn

Makes 1 serving

If you like your popcorn on the sweet side, this is your snack. To make this even more decadent, toast 2 tablespoons coconut flakes on the stovetop, then mix into your popcorn after it is popped. Melt ¼ dark chocolate bar in the microwave or on the stove, and drizzle on top.

Ingredients
1 tablespoon coconut oil
1 tablespoon honey or maple syrup
1 teaspoon cinnamon
2 tablespoons popcorn kernels
½ teaspoon salt

Directions
1. In a large pot over medium heat, combine the coconut oil, maple syrup, and cinnamon.
2. After the coconut oil has melted, add the kernels and cover, shaking the pot occasionally, until you hear popping. Turn heat off once there is a long time between the sounds of popping. Add the salt and shake to combine.

Trail Mix

Makes 1 serving

Here's the quickest snack you can prep. Consider making multiple servings of this delicious trail mix, so you have it on hand if the munchies hit.

Ingredients

1 small handful each of goji berries, raw almonds,
   raw cashews, and cacao nibs
1 teaspoon bee pollen

Directions

Place all ingredients in a baggie. Store in the pantry until ready to serve.

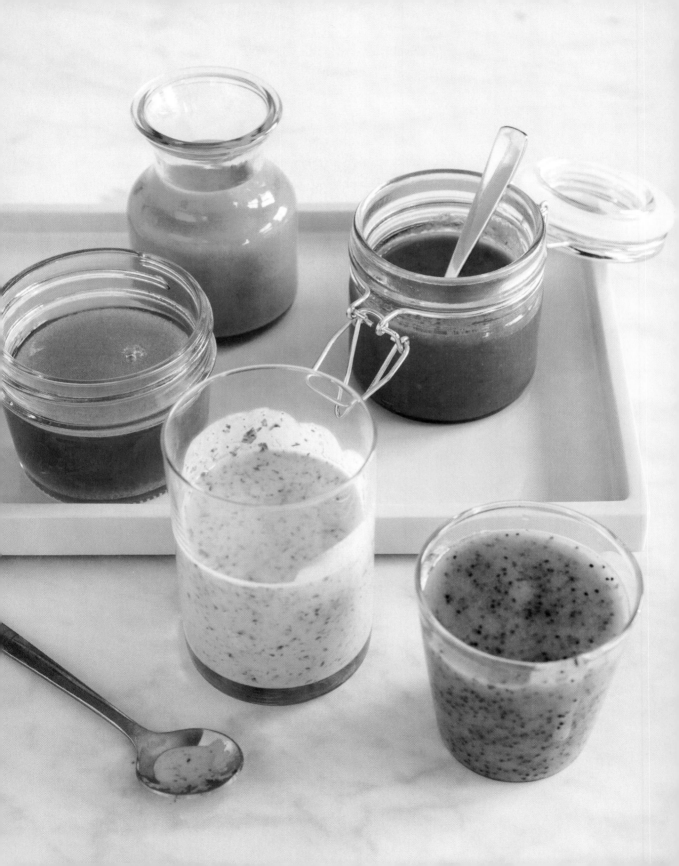

Salad Dressings

All of the dressings here are very effortless to make and they'll pair well with most recipes from the book. You can't go wrong when making a dressing—seriously! If you don't like one ingredient, swap it out for another. Also, feel free to use avocado oil or flaxseed oil instead of olive oil.

Each recipe makes 2 servings unless otherwise specified. Feel free to double or triple the recipes. Store them in the refrigerator, in individual containers or in larger ones.

Sweet and Sour Lemon Dressing

Ingredients
Juice of 1 lemon
2 tablespoons olive oil
1 tablespoon Dijon mustard
1 teaspoon turmeric
1 tablespoon honey
Pinch of cayenne (optional)

Directions

Place all ingredients in a blender or shaker, or mix by hand until fully combined. Separation is normal; stir or shake to recombine.

Sesame Tamari Dressing

Makes 3 servings

Ingredients

Juice of 1 orange
¼ cup rice wine vinegar
2 tablespoons liquid aminos or tamari
1 tablespoon toasted sesame oil
1 teaspoon honey
1 teaspoon finely grated ginger

Directions

Whisk orange juice, vinegar, liquid aminos or tamari, oil, honey, and ginger in a small bowl until the honey is fully incorporated.

Cilantro Tahini Dressing

Makes 3 servings

Ingredients

3 tablespoons tahini
2 tablespoons olive oil
¼ cup water
Juice of 1 lemon
1 small handful cilantro
1 garlic clove, crushed
Salt and pepper, to taste

Directions

Add all ingredients to a blender and blend until smooth. Season with salt and pepper.

Tomato Basil Vinaigrette

Makes 3-4 servings

Ingredients
3 sun-dried tomatoes
1 teaspoon crushed garlic
1 small handful basil leaves
2 tablespoons pine nuts
Juice of 1 lemon
2 tablespoons apple cider vinegar
½ teaspoon salt
Pinch of cayenne (optional)
1 teaspoon honey (optional)
¼ cup olive oil

Directions
Place all the ingredients except the oil in a blender. Blend for one minute, scraping down the sides as necessary. Slowly add in olive oil, stopping the blender occasionally and scraping down the sides.

Lemon Poppy Seed Dressing

Ingredients
½ cup olive oil
2 tablespoons lemon juice
1 teaspoon apple cider vinegar
1 tablespoon Dijon mustard
1 tablespoon poppy seeds
1 tablespoon honey or maple syrup

Directions
Place all ingredients into a mason jar or cup and mix by hand until well combined.

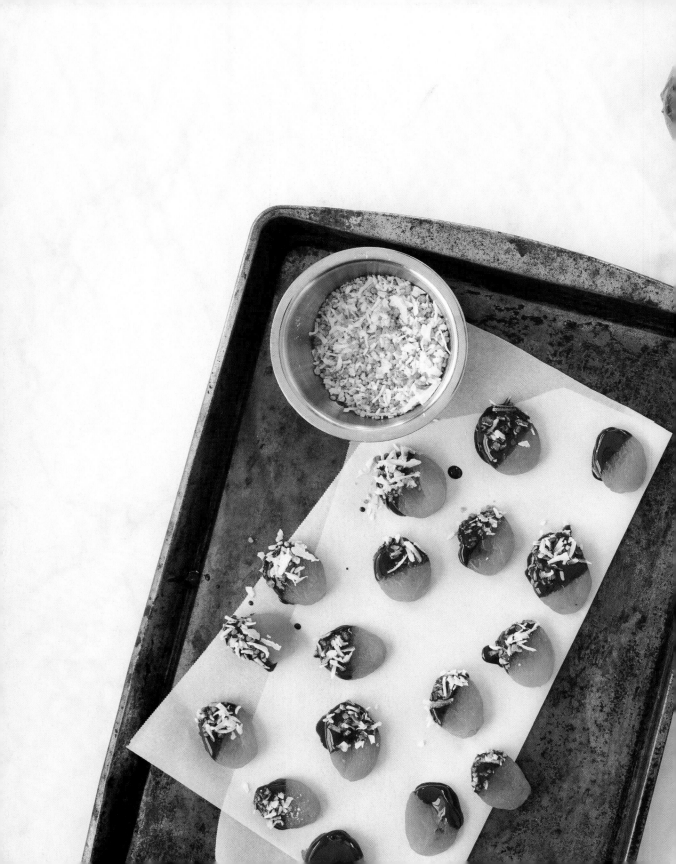

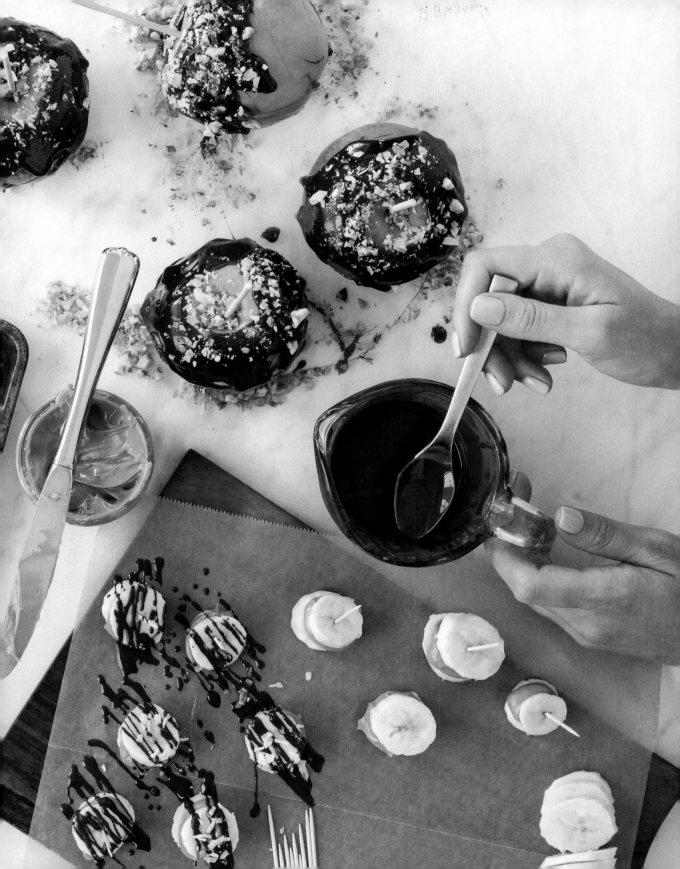

Desserts

Chocolate Pudding

Makes 1 to 2 servings

You won't believe the secret ingredient here: avocado. It gives the pudding a delicious mousse-like texture accented by honey, cacao powder, and other sweet flavors. If you like, top it with a small handful of chopped nuts, coconut flakes, bee pollen, or goji berries.

Ingredients
½ avocado
½ banana
1 to 2 tablespoons raw cacao powder
2 teaspoons raw honey or 1 Medjool date
¼ teaspoon vanilla extract
1 teaspoon Maple Cinnamon Almond Butter (page 191) (optional)
Pinch of salt

Directions
1. Place all ingredients in a blender and blend until smooth. Alternatively, mash the avocado by hand, and mix in the remainder of the ingredients.
2. Place in one or two containers. Refrigerate until ready to serve.

Chocolate-Covered Strawberries

Makes 4 servings

While this dessert might seem overly simple, most spend excess dollars for these during certain times of year. I adore the versatility of these and they've become a crowd-pleaser in my home because they are homemade.

Ingredients
1 pint strawberries
½ cup semi-sweet chocolate chips or 2 bars dark chocolate
1 cup almonds
½ cup coconut flakes
¼ cup crushed pistachios (optional)

Directions
1. Wash the strawberries well under running water. Pat them with paper towels and allow them to fully dry, out of the fridge. They do need to be dry, otherwise the chocolate will not stick to them.
2. Melt the chocolate in a small saucepan over medium-low heat, stirring constantly. Alternatively, place the chocolate in a small bowl and microwave it 30 seconds at a time, stirring in between, until the chocolate is melted. Be careful not to burn it.
3. Place the almonds in a plastic baggie and seal, then crush using the bottom of a cup. Add in coconut flakes and mix well. Spread this mixture out on a plate. Add pistachios if using.
4. Holding a strawberry by its leaves, dip each berry into the chocolate. Swirl the berries around until covered and gently shake off any excess chocolate.
5. Roll the strawberries in the almond-coconut mixture.
6. Place the strawberries in the refrigerator for 10 to 20 minutes in order to help the chocolate harden. They last about a week in the refrigerator.

Toffee Apples

Makes 4 desserts

Tired of crunching down on plain old apples? Not to worry, I've created the following decadent toffee apples that won't expand your waistline. (Just remember, though, moderation is key. This yummy snack contains a bit of coconut sugar and agave.)

Ingredients
3 tablespoons organic agave syrup or maple syrup
2 tablespoons coconut oil
2 tablespoons coconut sugar
¾ cup coconut milk
4 apples
4 wooden sticks
3 tablespoons chopped unsalted nuts

Directions
1. In a pan on high heat, cook the agave, coconut oil, and sugar until dissolved. Slowly add the coconut milk, stirring constantly.
2. Reduce to medium heat and cook, stirring frequently, for 15 minutes, or until thick.
3. While the caramel is thickening, wash and dry the apples. Insert the wooden sticks into the tops of the apples.
4. With a spoon, coat the apples in caramel and sprinkle the mixed nuts all over each apple. Place the toffee apples on a plate and place them in the refrigerator for at least one hour until the caramel sets (this may take longer), and serve.

Chocolate-Dipped Apricots with Coconut Flakes

Makes 1 serving

I'm a big fan of dried fruit, but I don't recommend eating it every day. Rather, think of it as a special treat and enjoy it occasionally. Adding dark chocolate and coconut flakes to dried fruit, as this recipe does, makes a gourmet-style dessert. You can switch out the apricots for dried mango, dried figs, or dried kiwi.

Ingredients
¼ cup dark chocolate chips
⅓ cup dried apricots
1 tablespoon coconut flakes (chopped more finely if you prefer)

Directions
1. Melt the chocolate in a small saucepan over medium-low heat, stirring constantly. Alternatively, place the chocolate in a small bowl and microwave it 30 seconds at a time, stirring in between, until the chocolate is melted. Be careful not to burn it.
2. Dip half of each apricot into the chocolate and place them on a baking sheet lined with parchment paper.
3. Sprinkle the coconut onto the chocolate. Let the apricots sit at room temperature until the chocolate hardens, or place in fridge to set them quicker.

Orange Hot Chocolate

When I was growing up, hot chocolate was one of my favorite things to drink during the winter months in Colorado. Here, I've updated the classic recipe so that it's both delicious *and* nutritious.

Ingredients

2 cups almond milk
1 teaspoon maca powder
3 tablespoons raw cacao powder
2 tablespoons honey
1 teaspoon vanilla extract
Zest of 1 orange

Directions

1. Place the milk in a saucepan and whisk in maca powder and cacao powder.
2. Bring to a light boil. Add honey, vanilla extract, and orange zest. Reduce heat to a simmer for two minutes. Strain and serve.

Chocolate PB Bites

Chocolate and peanut butter . . . I mean, what's better? These little bites are delectable, taste incredible, and are the perfect dessert to serve to friends or make with your kids. I recommend finding a peanut butter that is organic and has only peanuts listed in the ingredients.

Ingredients

1 banana
1 to 2 tablespoons peanut butter
1 teaspoon honey
¼ teaspoon vanilla extract
¼ teaspoon salt
2 tablespoons dark chocolate chips
1 tablespoon coconut flakes (optional)
1 teaspoon bee pollen (optional)

Directions

1. Peel the banana and cut into half-inch slices. Place the slices on a tray or plate lined with parchment paper.

2. Mix the peanut butter, honey, vanilla extract, and salt until well combined. Spread over half the banana slices. Place the other banana slices on top to create a tiny sandwich. Place a toothpick in the center and freeze for 20 minutes.

3. Place the chocolate in a small bowl and microwave it 30 seconds at a time, stirring in between, until the chocolate is melted. Be careful not to burn it.

4. Remove sandwiches from freezer and drizzle melted chocolate over each one. Sprinkle with coconut and bee pollen, if using. Return to the freezer and freeze for one hour or until banana is hard.

Raw No-Bake Vegan Cheesecake Slices

Makes 24 slices

It might seem like there are a lot of ingredients and work that goes into this recipe, but I promise you it's super simple—after you've made this once, you'll understand how easy it is to throw together. What takes the most time is soaking the cashews and freezing the mixture. Other than that, it's pretty foolproof.

Ingredients
½ cup almond meal
½ cup (packed) pitted Medjool dates, chopped
¾ teaspoon salt
½ teaspoon turmeric (optional)
1 cup raw cashews, soaked overnight
Juice of 1 lemon
¼ cup plus 1 tablespoon maple syrup
¼ cup coconut oil, melted
1 teaspoon vanilla extract
1 teaspoon maca powder (optional)
1 cup blueberries
½ cup strawberries
1 tablespoon maple syrup
1 tablespoon coconut flakes
1 tablespoon cacao nibs

Directions
1. Combine the almond meal, dates, ¼ teaspoon salt, and turmeric in a food processor. Pulse until a dough forms. Press the dough evenly into the bottom of a pan that has been lined with plastic wrap to fill the entire bottom, creating a thin base layer for your cheesecake.

2. Place the soaked cashews in a food processor along with the lemon juice, ¼ cup maple syrup, coconut oil, vanilla, maca powder, and ½ teaspoon salt. Blend until completely smooth, scraping down the sides occasionally. If the mixture is too thick, add small amounts of water until it has a creamy consistency.

3. Pour ¾ of the mixture onto the base layer, keeping the remaining ¼

mixture in the blender. Place the pan in the freezer for 10 minutes, which will make it so you can pour the next layer on top without them mixing.

4. To the remaining cheesecake mixture inside your blender, add the blueberries, blending until fully combined. Remove the cheesecake from the freezer and carefully add the blueberry layer on top, being careful not to mix the two layers. Use a spatula to evenly spread it out.

5. Place strawberries and maple syrup in a blender and blend until smooth. Drop the strawberry mixture by spoonfuls onto the top of the cheesecake, then use a toothpick or the tip of a knife to create a pattern by dragging it back and forth through the strawberry mixture. Top with coconut flakes and cacao nibs. Freeze at least two hours.

6. When ready to eat, remove from the freezer, slice, and let slices thaw for 10 to 15 minutes.

Coconut Dreamsicle Bliss Balls

Makes 20 to 25 balls (each snack/dessert serving is 4 to 5 balls)

These reminded me of those orange creamsicle pops I had as a kid, yet are elevated to a whole new level. Warning! They are incredibly scrumptous, so I recommend portioning them into small baggies to grab and go.

Ingredients

1 cup pitted Medjool dates
1 cup raw almonds
Zest of 1 orange
1 tablespoon orange juice
1 teaspoon lemon juice
½ teaspoon turmeric
½ teaspoon salt
½ teaspoon maca powder
¼ cup coconut flakes

Directions

1. In a food processor, blend the dates and almonds until well combined.
2. Add ½ of the orange zest plus the rest of the ingredients except the coconut flakes and blend until well combined. Transfer to a bowl to make it easier to handle the dough.
3. Put coconut flakes in the blender or food processor and process until finely chopped. Add the remaining orange zest and mix.
4. Roll the date-almond mixture into balls roughly one inch in diameter, then coat in the coconut mixture.
5. Freeze and remove when you're ready to eat.

Protein-Packed Paleo Brownies

Makes 8 brownies

For all you chocolate lovers out there, here is one of my favorite recipes. It's guilt-free, high in protein, and satisfying to your sweet tooth.

Ingredients
1 cup almond flour
¼ teaspoon salt
¼ teaspoon baking soda
½ teaspoon turmeric
1 teaspoon maca powder
4 ounces semisweet chocolate chips
7 Medjool dates, pitted
½ cup coconut oil
3 eggs
½ cup coconut sugar
½ cup cold water
½ cup coconut milk
1 teaspoon vanilla
Pinch of salt

Directions
1. Preheat the oven to 350 degrees.
2. In a food processor, pulse the almond flour, salt, baking soda, turmeric, and maca powder briefly until completely mixed.
3. Add chocolate and pulse briefly to create a grainy texture.
4. Add dates and pulse just until mixed.
5. Finally, pulse in the coconut oil and eggs until fully combined.
6. Grease an 8 × 8 baking dish with coconut oil and transfer the chocolate mixture to the dish. Smooth the top with a spatula.
7. Bake for 18 to 20 minutes, or until a knife inserted into the center comes out clean.
8. To make the caramel sauce, combine coconut sugar and water in a pan over medium-low heat and cook, stirring constantly, until completely

dissolved. Let bubble 2 to 3 minutes. Pour in coconut milk, stirring constantly. Simmer on low heat for 10 to 15 minutes, stirring occasionally.

9. Remove from heat and stir in the vanilla and salt. Let cool. Pour the sauce on the brownies once they are cooled.

10. To store, refrigerate the brownies.

CHAPTER 16

Meal Prep Beyond the 28 Days

Congratulations—you have completed my 28-day meal prep plan. Now that you've crossed the finish line, what happens next?

I've found through years of dieting that it's easier to stick to a plan when you know exactly what's on your shopping list, what to eat each day, and how often to eat. But when the plan ends, you worry about slipping back into bad habits. Rest assured: if you followed everything faithfully for four weeks, you're well on your way to making meal prep and healthy eating a lifestyle. Psychologists say it takes 21 days to form new habits. You've been meal prepping for 28 days. So, psychologically speaking, you've cemented good habits and are on your way to being a lifetime meal prepper—and one who is beautifully fit and healthy.

The plan you've just followed changes your lifestyle effectively so that you'll automatically maintain your weight loss and all the benefits that go with it. You never had to count calories or points or grams of anything. You just portioned out real food, enjoyed it, and lost weight in the process. You've learned what proper portion sizes look like—knowledge you can use to help you shed more weight or keep off what you've already lost. You know that you're capable of overcoming emotional overeating. I doubt you'll ever slip back to eating second and third helpings, or bingeing, as long as you continue to prep in the manner I've outlined here and follow my tips for emotional eating.

I'm not down on other diets, and I'm not saying they don't work. What I'm saying is that you have to shift your mindset about the foods you eat, and *why* you eat them. Remember, even this plan is not a "diet"; it is a way of life that you can tailor to your personal preferences.

The best way to enjoy lifelong results and feel the healthiest and sexiest you ever have is by continuing the good habits you've put into place over the last 28 days: Focus on plant foods. Plan and prep your foods. Enjoy super ingredients. Remember that food is your friend, not your enemy.

Assess Your Progress

To capitalize on your results and to prevent yourself from slipping back into old habits, pull out your journal and answer the following questions:

- What was the most important lesson you learned during the 28 days?
- What were your favorite breakfasts, lunches, dinners, and snacks? Why did you like them so much?
- What are the key foods you must prep—without fail—to experience success each week?
- What is motivating you to continue a healthy lifestyle (how you look, how you feel, how you approach life, and so forth)?
- Have you found that meal prepping eases your stress, curbs emotional eating, or both?

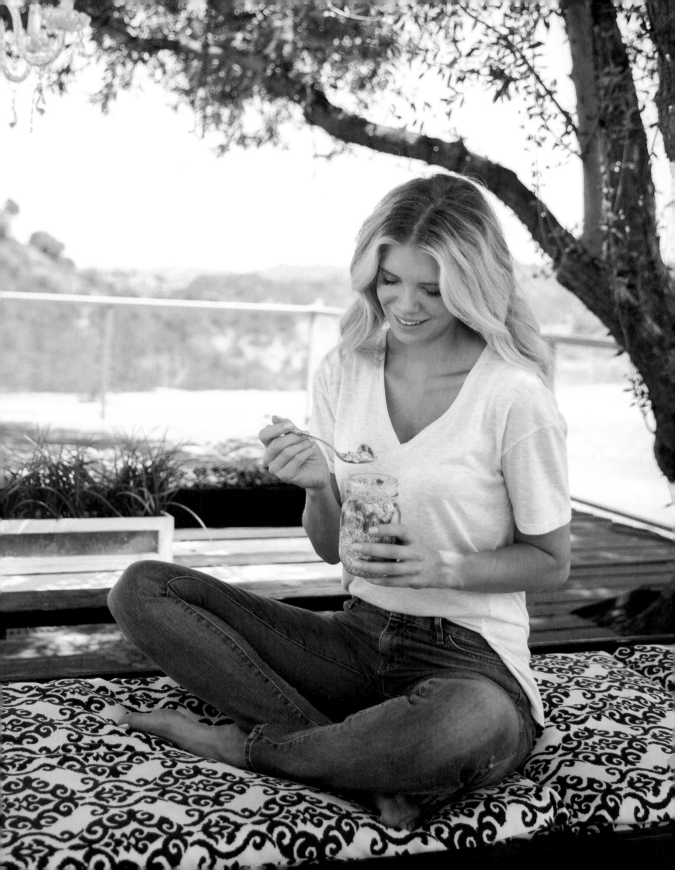

- If you could teach someone else about what you learned, what would you share?
- How will you set yourself up for success when you travel?
- How will you plan for parties, meals at restaurants, or when you might feel tempted by a food you'll later feel guilty about eating?

Putting pen to paper and focusing on these triumphs is one of the best ways to stay on track. Stay positive and constructive here; this is not a time to beat yourself up. Focusing on the positive will make you feel successful, and you can build on those successes. On days when you don't feel so great, read back over your answers to keep your drive afire.

Strategies Going Forward

As I've mentioned, I used to be a perpetual dieter. But no more. I just eat healthy, unprocessed foods most of the time. I'm dedicated to meal prep because I know it works and keeps me on track. Along the way, I've learned a lot of strategies that work in the long term.

- Let go of trying to be perfect with your diet—and the guilt that comes with less-than-perfect performance. Instead, focus on what makes you feel good. Eating a piece of chocolate cake when out with friends to celebrate a birthday can be a beautiful thing, because at that moment it's not about the food, it's about sharing the experience.
- Each week, write down recipes from this plan that you'd like to enjoy in the future, such as the Quinoa Lime Fruit Salad or Collard Wraps, and put the necessary ingredients on your shopping list.
- Choose one new recipe a week to try if you're feeling adventurous. This is the best way to continue this new healthy lifestyle. It keeps things fun and prevents you from getting bored and going back to old habits.
- Invite friends over and cook a meal from the 28-day plan.

- When dining, make choices from the menu that include various super fruits, vegetables, and grains; don't be afraid to ask for modifications. This way, you can create your own super meals at restaurants.

- Focus on eating three or more colors at each meal; this is the quickest way to stop counting calories, lose weight, and become nutritionally healthy for life.

- Create a calendar each week that outlines when you will meal prep and what days you'll eat your prepped meals. Allow a few meals each week for things like business lunches and dinners with friends.

- Choose one day a week when you will eat a favorite food (remember, no guilt here, so we're not calling it a cheat meal) and stick with that one meal.

- Write down what you are grateful for each day, either when you wake up or when you go to sleep. Your thoughts have a powerful effect on your lifestyle.

My Meal Prep Plan Is Adaptable

Go forward with the knowledge that every recipe in this book can be modified to fit your lifestyle and how you like to eat. If you are a vegan, for example, simply modify recipes that include something you wouldn't normally eat. If a recipe calls for eggs in baking, use chia seeds soaked in water as a substitute. If you like to eat meat, choose quality over quantity and add in one or two pieces of the best quality you can get, in place of any plant-based protein. Just because a recipe might call for something specific does not mean you need to stick to it as written. This is important because I have many friends who see a recipe that looks delicious but then realize it has honey in it and suddenly they won't even consider it anymore. The simple swap here would be to use agave, maple syrup, or coconut syrup instead. The great thing about cooking, and I hope you've learned this throughout the book, is that you can adjust anything to fit your needs. If you absolutely want more fish or chicken in the plan, then add it to one more meal a week. The same goes for removing an animal product and adding something vegan or vegetarian.

Prepping Support

Healthy eating can be tough, and it can also be lonely. To help you in the future, it's important to have support from your family and friends.

Receiving social support is vital in motivating us to lose weight and keep it off, says a 2014 study from the University of Illinois at Urbana-Champaign. The researchers conducted focus groups with twenty-three women about a year and a half after they completed a weight-loss program to determine which factors helped or hindered dieters' success. While all of the women who participated lost a significant amount of weight on the program, many were unsuccessful at maintaining the weight loss after the program ended.

The women who kept the weight off indicated that a high level of social support, especially from someone who was going through the same experience, was critical to their success. So if you can find that one friend who has the same goals or can just hold you accountable, it's really beneficial.

How do you go about that?

I have a few tips and tricks that have worked for me. But before I share, I want to caution you against judging others for not living the same lifestyle as you or wanting to make a change like you are. You can serve as a guiding light for others—without passing judgment.

Your loved ones mean the world to you and you want them to be full of energy and eating foods that will nourish their body. It can be incredibly tough to watch them do things that you know are not good for them. Have you found yourself in this situation?

The only way to truly change someone else's habits is to change yours first. No one likes being told what to do, but people are much more willing to make a change if they can follow someone else's example.

A quick story: A previous partner of mine didn't live the same lifestyle as I did. This bothered me. I got very upset when I saw him eating lots of meat, not getting enough exercise, not drinking enough water, and overall just not taking care of his body. Deep down, I knew that if he made a few minor changes, he'd feel so much better and our relationship would grow.

At first I nagged him about it. How did that work? Not well. It caused lots of fights.

I decided to let go of trying to control his behavior. I passed no judgment; I did not nag. Instead, I'd gently ask him if he wanted lemon water in the morning, to go on beach walks at night (rather than insist on gym workouts), or get involved with meal prep work for dinners. At first he was reluctant, but because I let him choose, he gradually got on board. He changed a lot of his habits, and it made me so happy to see that he was starting to appreciate a healthier lifestyle.

What I learned is that you can't change someone's habits, nor should you try. Change is up to them. All you can do is set a good example. Be the person who inspires those around you and makes them want to change because they see how wonderful you look and feel.

Once you feel a family member or loved one is on the same path as you are, here are some additional pieces of advice:

- Have your loved ones look over the meal plan each week and see what recipes look interesting to them. Put them on your planning calendar to prep and cook these meals together.
- Cook breakfast for your partner from the plan on a Saturday or Sunday morning and surprise them in bed.
- Ask your friends or loved ones if they'd be willing to do one week of the plan with you, with no pressure to go further.
- See if your family members or partner would like to eat *only* the dinners from the plan with you; this makes it seem very approachable.
- Organize a group of your co-workers to do the plan; I suggest creating a group text thread or private Facebook group to keep each other accountable.
- Create a system of non-food rewards for everyone who completes the plan with you.
- Ask your family members or partner to help you meal prep on

Sunday, with no judgment if they don't want to do the actual plan—at least they are helping you meal prep!

- Prep an extra smoothie in the mornings, or an additional serving of any other breakfast, and leave it for your partner or family member. Do this repeatedly for a few days; it might encourage them to enjoy these recipes. Keep doing this until it becomes a habit for them.

- Don't dine in front of the TV. Even if you're eating a different meal from your family, make sure everyone still sits down at the dinner table. And put away the phones! Conversation during meals makes us slow down and increases our digestion.

- Have your kids (or even your hubby!) help you spiralize zucchini, and give them jobs like washing the fruits and vegetables, putting items in a blender, and garnishing smoothies.

- Make meal prep and cooking fun. Don't allow these activities to become a drag. Instead listen to music, dance in the kitchen with your kids, and make your partner feel loved while you prepare the meal.

- Show appreciation and thanks for even a little support and involvement. You don't need to get their full commitment, but every little bit counts.

Continue to listen to your body and give it what it needs, and you will feel the best you ever have. There is no right or wrong, it's what works best for you. You are the master of your own beautiful body and how you feel.

ACKNOWLEDGMENTS

Before I thank anyone, I'd like to really thank the chocolate that I'm eating right now . . . because without it, I wouldn't be a very happy girl.

So here's to the food we enjoy and learning to live a more balanced life while eating chocolate and green smoothies!

With that, I thank the following people:

My mother and Jim, who always give copies of my books to their friends, showing off how proud they are of me. I love you both and really do appreciate your love and support. I can't wait to talk about this book at your next summer party!

My father, who is probably off traveling the world and cycling his 100-mile rides in Europe. Thank you for challenging me to do things outside of my comfort zone. Although I can be stubborn about the things you say (a lot has changed from my being a kid, clearly), I love that you help me grow and become a better human.

My agents, Scott Hoffman and Steve Troha, for being with me in the journey from my first proposal a few years ago, to the publisher meetings, and now to my second book. I am thankful to have you both by my side. I hope we can continue the celebrations we had in NYC after the initial meetings and look forward to the success of this and more books in the future.

Maggie, my dear Maggie. You are just truly an amazing human, and I am beyond thankful that our paths crossed. Thank you for believing in me, sharing your stories, and making me laugh even when times were stressful. I look forward to many more acknowledgments with you in them!

Random House, which made my dream of becoming an author come true with my first book, *The 5-Day Real Food Detox*. My team at Ballantine took a chance on me, and I am beyond appreciative for this opportunity. The things we dream about can actually come true!

Sara Weiss, my editor, Joe Perez, Anna Bauer, Diane Hobbing, Ted Allen, Colleen Nuccio, Emily Isayeff, and Elana Seplow-Jolley! Thank you for your amazing guidance, editing, and assistance throughout this project—all of which made the book better than I could ever imagine. I am beyond excited to share this book with you after all your hard work. It really does take a village to make a book like this happen, and you all have been rock stars.

My photo shoot team: Pam McLean, thank you for taking my vision and turning it into reality. I am beyond grateful for your hard work and beautiful work. Tuan Tran, thank you for your help with the shoot, helping Pam out and making sure everything was executed to perfection. John Galang, I'm so glad that we worked together and that you were able to style my food with no questions asked despite my crazy ways. Raquel Alessi, it was wonderful to work with you, listen to your stories, and have you assist on the book.

All my friends who have helped me throughout the years, listened to my stories, helped me through the low moments, celebrated the highs, and supported me in my journey. I love you all!

EC—you've taught me a lot, guided me, and while some questions might never be answered, thank you for being a big influence on my life. So here's to Jaks and all the crazy experiences in between.

Kerri—You have been my cheerleader for years now. I'm so beyond appreciative that your stalking and the app brought us together (I laugh because people will be wondering what I mean here, LOL!). You've been such an inspiring person to have in my life and I am just astounded at how I lucked out to have a friend like you. Here's to online banter, London, LA, SF, Africa, and all the rest of our adventures! Love you!

And all of *you* for reading this book. Without you, my incredibly amazing community, I wouldn't be writing books like this. Thank you for

ACKNOWLEDGMENTS

being on this journey with me. Together, we can inspire those around us and help make this world a better place. I encourage you to share this book with your friends and family, because finding community with those you care about will have a greater impact on your health and happiness . . . and hey, it's much easier to stick to a plan when you do it with others!

Finally, everyone I didn't mention here: just know that I love you, even if we haven't met. I am so incredibly grateful to everyone I've encountered along my path and I look forward to whatever comes next. You all inspire me to be a better person, put out awesome content, and help people live their best lives.

Until the next book . . .

Tons of love,

Nikki

APPENDIX A

Bonus Meal Prep: Meals That Freeze with Ease

No matter how dedicated I am to meal prepping, I've had some days when my best-laid plans go out the window. That's why I advise stocking your freezer with prepped foods for emergencies. Freezing foods is also a great solution if you have a hectic lifestyle.

Here are my favorite freezable meals that you can find in my freezer at any given time.

Breads and Breakfast Dishes

Gluten-Free Brown Bread

Missing your morning toast, or a chunk of bread with your soup? Well, don't worry—this tasty bread recipe will be sure to please.

Ingredients

450 g gluten-free brown bread flour
½ teaspoon salt
2 tablespoons rapid-rise yeast
350 ml of warm almond milk
1 tablespoon vinegar
1 tablespoon honey, preferably organic
2 eggs
6 tablespoons coconut oil

Directions

1. Preheat the oven to 350 degrees.
2. Mix the flour, salt, and yeast together.
3. In a large bowl, beat together the milk, vinegar, honey, and eggs.
4. Add the flour mixture to the milk mixture to form a sticky dough. Continue mixing while adding the oil slowly.
5. Place the dough in an oiled 1 kg loaf pan, cover, and set aside in a warm place for 1 hour to rise.
6. Once the loaf has risen, bake it for 40 to 45 minutes.
7. Remove from the oven and allow to cool.
8. Wrap tightly and freeze.

Banana Bread

Need to do something with those overripe bananas that are about to go bad? Banana bread to the rescue.

Ingredients

2 very ripe bananas, mashed
2 eggs
2 tablespoons coconut oil, melted
1 tablespoon vanilla extract
1 ½ teaspoons baking powder
1 cup almond flour
1 tablespoon cinnamon
½ cup coconut flour
½ teaspoon salt
1 handful chopped walnuts
1 handful dark chocolate chips (optional)

Directions

1. Preheat oven to 350 degrees.
2. Mix together the bananas, eggs, coconut oil, and vanilla extract.
3. In a separate bowl, combine the baking powder, almond flour, cinnamon, coconut flour, and salt. Stir the dry ingredients into the wet ingredients.
4. Stir in walnuts and chocolate chips.
5. Grease your loaf pan (you used for the Paleo Bread, see p. 189) with coconut oil, then add the batter.
6. Bake 30 to 35 minutes, or until a knife inserted into the center comes out clean. Allow to cool. To store, wrap tightly and freeze.

Guilt-Free Crepes

This recipe is super easy to make and it's a high-protein and energy-boosting breakfast option. Usually I put some frozen berries in a dish and microwave for 30 seconds until they are soft and juicy to pour on top of my crepes. I also sprinkle a little xylitol on top, which is my favorite zero-calorie sweetener. If you'd like to save some money, making your own oat flour is very easy. Take 1 cup oats and blitz on high in your high-speed blender until flour forms.

Ingredients
1 cup oat flour
2 large eggs
1 tablespoon agave
¼ teaspoon vanilla
¼ cup water
1 tablespoon coconut oil

Directions
1. Place all ingredients except the coconut oil in a blender and blend well.
2. Heat the coconut oil in a skillet or crepe pan on medium heat. Pour about ¼ cup batter into the center of the pan and spread it around so that the crepe is very thin. Cook for about 2 minutes, or until the bottom of the crepe is brown. Flip the crepe over and cook on the other side. Repeat this process for the remaining 3 crepes.
3. Let crepes cool on a plate. To freeze, layer the crepes between sheets of waxed paper and wrap in plastic wrap.
4. When ready to serve, let the crepes thaw, reheat, and top with fresh berries.

Two-Ingredient Pancakes Plus

These pancakes not only are delicious and healthy but also are packed full of protein and are low in carbs. They make the perfect breakfast, snack, or post-workout meal. The "plus" stands for protein powder (I use the Just Add Water brand), but it's optional here. Top with fresh berries, 1 tablespoon of Greek yogurt or coconut yogurt, and a sprinkle of cinnamon. I often add chopped mint for extra flavor and nutrition.

Ingredients
1 ripe banana, mashed
2 eggs
1 scoop protein powder (optional)
1 tablespoon coconut oil

Directions

1. Combine all ingredients except the coconut oil and mix very well. (I use a blender.)

2. Heat the coconut oil in a skillet on medium heat. Add batter by large spoonfuls to the pan.

3. Cook 1 to 2 minutes. Flip the pancakes after they bubble. Cook the other side.

4. Transfer to a plate; allow to cool. Wrap tightly and freeze.

5. When ready to serve, let the pancakes thaw, then reheat.

Pumpkin Delight Donuts

Yes, you can make your own donuts, and you can make them healthy. Most commercial donuts are fried and contain all sorts of hidden ingredients. These are baked, and you control what goes in them. An added bonus is that they're gluten-free. Try spreading these with my Maple Cinnamon Almond Butter (page 191).

Ingredients

5 eggs
½ cup coconut milk
½ cup maple syrup
¼ cup coconut oil, and some for greasing
1 teaspoon vanilla extract
½ cup canned pumpkin
¾ cup almond flour
½ cup coconut flour
1 teaspoon baking soda
1 teaspoon pumpkin pie spice
Pinch of salt

Directions

1. Preheat the oven to 350 degrees.
2. Place the eggs, coconut milk, maple syrup, coconut oil, and vanilla in a blender and blend. Add the remaining ingredients and blend until smooth.
3. Lightly grease a donut pan with coconut oil and pour the mixture into the molds, filling them ¾ full.
4. Bake for 17 to 20 minutes. For a moister center, bake only 17 minutes; for normal cake texture, bake for 20 minutes.
5. Remove from the oven. Allow to cool. Wrap each donut tightly and freeze until ready to eat, then thaw.

Double Chocolate Muffins

These muffins are a wonderfully tasty breakfast or snack. Plus they freeze beautifully, and thaw quickly. The kidney beans may seem like an unusual ingredient, but they fill in for flour to create a high-fiber, yummy muffin.

Ingredients
3 eggs
1 can (15 ounces) red kidney beans, drained and rinsed
3 tablespoons coconut oil, plus some for greasing
1 tablespoon açai powder (optional)
¼ teaspoon vanilla extract
½ cup raw cacao powder
½ cup agave syrup or honey
½ teaspoon baking powder

Directions
1. Preheat oven to 350 degrees.
2. Place all ingredients in a blender or food processor and blend on low, scraping sides as necessary until combined.
3. Lightly coat a muffin tin with coconut oil. Pour mixture into cups, filling each halfway.
4. Bake for 20 minutes. The inside should still be slightly gooey (stick a knife in to check). Let rest a few minutes before removing from the tin. Cool completely. Wrap each muffin tightly and freeze.

Entrées

Mexican Bean Soup

Here's a true super meal in soup form. It incorporates seven super ingredients in one pot—which means it's loaded with fiber, antioxidants, and phytochemicals. But beyond the nutrition, this soup is tangy and flavorful. You'll probably want a second helping, but it's so filling, you might not need one.

Ingredients

1 teaspoon olive oil
1 red onion, finely chopped
2 to 3 garlic cloves, minced
2 carrots, peeled and diced
1 red pepper, seeded and diced
1 teaspoon cayenne
1 teaspoon ground cumin
10 fluid ounces water
½ vegetable stock cube
1 can (14 ounces) diced tomatoes
1 can (15 ounces) red kidney beans or black beans, drained and rinsed
Salt and pepper, to taste

Directions

1. In a medium-sized pan, heat the oil and sauté the onion, garlic, and carrots until the onions are translucent and the carrots are tender. Then add the red pepper, cayenne, and cumin, stirring to combine. Cook another minute.

2. Measure 1 ¼ cups of water into a pan. Add the stock cube and bring to a boil, making sure the cube dissolves.

3. Stir in the onion mixture and the tomatoes and cook for 10 minutes.

4. Add the beans and cook for another 5 minutes. Season with salt and pepper.

5. Portion into separate freezable containers and freeze.

Lentil Veggie Stew

Lentils are an excellent source of fiber and easy to cook (no soaking time required!) This recipe serves up a hearty stew, and you won't miss the meat.

Ingredients
2 tablespoons olive oil
1 onion, chopped
4 large cloves garlic, minced
½ cup balsamic vinegar
4 cups vegetable stock
2 cups lentils, rinsed
2 carrots, thinly sliced
2 stalks celery, chopped (including leaves)
1 large red bell pepper, seeded and diced
½ teaspoon dried oregano
½ teaspoon dried basil
Salt and pepper, to taste

Directions

1. Heat oil in a large soup pot over medium-high heat. Add onion and garlic and cook 2 to 3 minutes, or until translucent. Add the vinegar and allow to lightly bubble.

2. Add 4 cups stock along with the lentils, carrots, celery, and bell pepper. Bring to a boil then reduce heat to a simmer and cover with a lid, cooking for 15 minutes.

3. Stir in oregano and basil. Lower heat to medium. Cover and simmer for 1 hour. Season to taste with salt and pepper.

4. Portion into freezable containers and freeze.

Beet and Asparagus Soup

This soup takes just a few minutes to make. You can double the batch and have enough leftovers for a few meals. Or freeze it, of course! If you're going vegan, leave out the shredded chicken and add in some tofu, tempeh, or cooked buckwheat groats.

Ingredients
3 fresh beets, peeled
2 cups vegetable stock
1 bunch fresh asparagus, chopped
1 cup shredded cooked chicken (optional)

Directions
1. Place the beets in a pot, cover with 1 to 2 cups water, and bring to a boil. Cook on medium-high heat for 20 minutes, or until tender.
2. Add the vegetable stock and asparagus. Cook 3 minutes, or until soft.
3. Pour the mixture into a blender or food processor. Blend until creamy. Season with salt, pepper, and any additional super herbs or spices, as desired.
4. Add the chicken, if using, and heat through.
5. Portion into separate freezable containers and freeze.

Vegan Quiche

I love quiche for breakfast, brunch, lunch, and dinner. It's perfect for any meal. I recently learned how to create this vegan quiche, and it's wonderful. I don't even miss its more fattening, calorie-laden counterpart.

Ingredients
½ small onion, chopped
1 tablespoon olive oil
1 pound silken tofu
1 tablespoon nutritional yeast flakes
½ teaspoon garlic powder
¼ teaspoon dry mustard
¼ teaspoon white pepper
¼ teaspoon salt
½ cup shredded vegan cheese
1 frozen vegan pie shell, 9- to 10-inch diameter

Directions
1. Preheat oven to 400 degrees.
2. In a small skillet, sauté onion in olive oil on medium heat until onion is translucent. Remove from heat and set aside.
3. Puree the tofu, nutritional yeast flakes, garlic powder, mustard, pepper, and salt in a blender. Mix in the vegan cheese and sautéed onions.
4. Pour the tofu mixture into the pie shell, place it on a cookie sheet, and bake for 10 to 15 minutes, or until the crust is brown and a knife inserted in the center comes out clean.
5. Remove from the oven and allow it to cool. Wrap it well and freeze until you are ready to serve. To reheat the frozen quiche, do not let it thaw; just pop it right into the oven.

Quinoa Chili

Here's a superfood-filled twist on chili that you'll love.

Ingredients

1 tablespoon olive oil
1 onion, finely chopped
2 cloves garlic, minced
1 jalepeño
1 green bell pepper, chopped
4 large tomatoes, chopped
2 cans (15 ounces each) black beans, drained and rinsed
1 can (15 ounces) kidney beans, drained and rinsed
1 jar (28 ounces) chunky salsa
1 cup water
1 cup quinoa, rinsed and cooked per package directions
1 tablespoon chili powder
2 teaspoons ground cumin
Salt and pepper, to taste

Directions

1. In a large stockpot over medium heat, warm the olive oil. Add the onion, garlic, jalepeño, green bell pepper, and tomatoes, and cook, stirring, until the onions are soft, about 5 to 7 minutes.

2. Add the black beans, kidney beans, salsa, and 1 cup water. Stir in the quinoa. Add the chili powder and cumin, and season with salt and pepper. Over high heat, bring the mixture to a boil. Reduce the heat to medium-low and simmer uncovered, stirring occasionally, until thickened, about 35 to 40 minutes. Adjust seasonings as needed.

Paleo Meatballs

These meatballs taste delicious, especially served with spiralized zucchini (subbing for pasta) and your favorite marinara sauce.

Ingredients

1 onion, chopped
8 ounces lean ground turkey or buffalo meat
1 tablespoon honey
1 egg, beaten
Handful of arugula, finely chopped
½ teaspoon cayenne
Salt and pepper, to taste
1 tablespoon olive oil

Directions

1. In a bowl, use your hands to mix together the onion, meat, honey, egg, arugula, and cayenne. Season with salt and pepper.
2. Form the mixture into 8 meatballs.
3. Heat olive oil in a small skillet on medium heat. Add meatballs and sauté with the lid on until they are cooked through, about 5 to 8 minutes.
4. Remove from heat and allow to cool. Transfer the meatballs to a freezable container and freeze. When ready to serve, thaw and reheat the meatballs and serve.

Desserts

Chocolate Banana Sorbet

Enjoy this frosty treat on a hot night. It takes seconds to whip up and stores wonderfully in the freezer.

Ingredients
2 ripe bananas, peeled, sliced, and frozen overnight
2 teaspoons cacao powder
1 tablespoon honey

Directions
1. Place all ingredients in a blender and blend until thick and creamy.
2. Pour mixture into separate freezable containers and freeze. When ready to serve, allow each serving to thaw slightly.

Raspberry Vanilla Cheesecake

I love to make raw cheesecakes because they are super easy and incredibly delicious.

Ingredients

½ cup nuts or seeds (walnuts, almonds, Brazil nuts, or pumpkin seeds)
½ cup pitted Medjool dates
Pinch of salt
1 ½ cups raw cashews, soaked at least 4 hours
Juice of 2 lemons
1 to 2 teaspoons vanilla extract
⅓ cup coconut oil
⅓ cup honey or agave syrup
1 cup fresh raspberries

Directions

1. Place the nuts or seeds, dates, and salt in a food processor and process until a dough forms. Press the mixture evenly into the bottom of a 9-inch springform pan creating the crust for your cheesecake.

2. In a food processor, combine cashews, lemon juice, vanilla, coconut oil, and honey. Blend until completely smooth, scraping down the sides as necessary.

3. Pour ⅔ of the mixture over the crust, smoothing with a spoon. Leave ⅓ of the mix in the food processor and add the raspberries; blend until smooth. Pour over first layer.

4. Cover and place the cheesecake in freezer. When ready to serve, remove from freezer and let it partially thaw.

Tropical Treat Ice Cream

I have a tropical treat for you: piña coladas in ice cream form! It's a refreshing combo of banana, coconut, and vanilla ice cream—so easy and delicious that you'll want to keep your freezer stocked with this dessert.

Ingredients

1 banana, peeled, sliced, and frozen for at least an hour
3 unsalted raw Brazil nuts
1 tablespoon goji berries
1 tablespoon coconut oil
1 teaspoon vanilla extract
1 tablespoon cacao nibs (optional)

Directions

1. Place the banana, nuts, berries, coconut oil, and vanilla in a blender or food processor. Process 2 minutes, scraping down the sides occasionally, until smooth.

2. Add the cacao nibs and do one last quick blitz to roughly chop them.

3. Portion the mixture into separate freezable containers and freeze.

Coco-Pops

What I love about homemade popsicles is that they contain simple, healthy ingredients—and taste better than anything you can buy at the grocery store. Plus, they take just minutes to make. Mine are simple, delicious, and contain no additives.

Ingredients
1 banana, peeled and sliced
2 tablespoons honey
½ cup coconut milk
5 strawberries, hulled and chopped
¼ cup blueberries

Directions
1. Place the banana, honey, and coconut milk in a blender and blend.
2. Pour this mixture into popsicle molds. Divide the strawberries and blueberries among the molds, pushing them into the middle and on the sides of the molds.
3. Freeze. When you're ready to enjoy these, simply run the mold under hot water for a few minutes to make it easy to remove the popsicle from the mold.

Green Tea Ice Cream

Can ice cream ever be healthy? Yes—if you make it this way, with high-antioxidant matcha, which is green tea powder. Beyond its nutritional merits, this ice cream is super delicious. Top with sliced almonds, chopped mint, or—my favorite—cacao nibs, for that chocolate chip feel.

Ingredients

2 ripe bananas, peeled, sliced, and frozen
1 small handful mint
1 teaspoon matcha
¼ cup coconut milk (optional)
1 tablespoon honey or agave syrup (optional)

Directions

1. Place all ingredients in a blender and blend until smooth and creamy.

2. At this point, the mixture will resemble soft serve, and it's totally delectable. If you would like a more traditional ice cream texture, place it in a bowl and put it back in the freezer for another 30 minutes.

APPENDIX B

References

Al-Alawi, R. A., et al. 2017. Date palm tree (*Phoenix dactylifera* L.): natural products and therapeutic options. *Frontiers in Plant Science* 8: 845.

ANI. 2009. Alcohol consumption linked to "pound a month" weight gain: UK study. *Hindustan Times,* December 1, online.

Bae, J., et al. 2015. Fennel (*Foeniculum vulgare*) and fenugreek (*Trigonella foenum-graecum*) tea drinking suppresses subjective short-term appetite in overweight women. *Clinical Nutrition Research* 4: 168–174.

Barreca, D., et al. 2017. Flavanones: Citrus phytochemical with health-promoting properties. *Biofactors*, May 12, online.

Beezhold, B., et al. 2015. Vegans report less stress and anxiety than omnivores. *Nutritional Neuroscience* 18: 289–296.

Bryan, J., Calvaresi, E., et al. Associations between dietary intake of folate and vitamins B-12 and B-6 and self-reported cognitive function and psychological well-being in Australian men and women in midlife. *Journal of Nutrition, Health, and Aging* 8: 226–232.

Butt, M. S., et al. 2013. Anti-oncogenic perspectives of spices/herbs: A comprehensive review. *EXCLI Journal* 12: 1043–1065.

Chang, R. C., and So, K. F. 2008. Use of anti-aging herbal medicine,

Lycium barbarum, against aging-associated diseases. What do we know so far? *Cellular and Molecular Neurobiology* 28: 643–652.

Cui, T., et al. 2015. A urologist's guide to ingredients found in top-selling nutraceuticals for men's sexual health. *Journal of Sexual Medicine* 12: 2105–2117.

Denisow, B., and Denisow-Pietrzyk, M. Biological and therapeutic properties of bee pollen: a review. *Journal of the Science of Food and Agriculture* 96: 4303–4309.

De Souza Ferreira, C., et al. 2015. Effect of chia seeds (*Salvia hispanica* L.) consumption on cardiovascular risk factors in humans: a systemic review. *Nutricion Hospitalaria* 32: 1909–1918.

Dreher, M. L., and Davenport, A.J. 2013. Hass avocado composition and potential health effects. *Critical Reviews in Food Science and Nutrition* 53: 738–750.

Dzoyem, J. P., et al. 2014. The 15-lipoxygenase inhibitory, antioxidant, antimycobacterial activity and cytotoxicity of fourteen ethnomedicinally used African spices and culinary herbs. *Journal of Ethnopharmocolgy* 156: 1–8.

Fresan, U., et al. 2016. Substitution models of water for other beverages, and the incidence of obesity and weight gain in the SUN cohort. *Nutrients* 31: E688.

Gimenez-Bastida, J. A., and Zielinski, H. 2015. Buckwheat as a functional food and its effects on health. *Journal of Agricultural and Food Chemistry* 63: 7896–7913.

Giovanni, M., et al. 2010. Symposium overview: Do we all eat breakfast and is it important? *Critical Reviews in Food Science and Nutrition* 50: 97–99.

Harvard Health Letter. 2013. Skipping breakfast hurts heart health, says Harvard study. *Harvard Health Letter* 38: 8.

Hooshmand, B., et al. 2012. Associations between serum homocysteine, holotranscobalamin, folate and cognition in the elderly: a longitudinal study. *Journal of Internal Medicine* 271: 204–212.

Hosseini, S. M., et al. 2013. Nutritional and medical applications of spirulina microalgae. *Mini Reviews in Medicinal Chemistry* 13: 1231–1237.

Khan, M. S., et al. 2015. Chromatographic analysis of wheatgrass extracts. *Journal of Pharmacy and Bioallied Sciences* 7: 267–271.

Khan, N., et al. 2013. Fisetin: a dietary antioxidant for health promotion. *Antioxidants and Redox Signaling* 19: 151–162.

Kim, S.J., and de Souza, R. J. 2016. Effects of dietary pulse consumption on body weight: A systematic review and meta-analysis of randomized controlled trials. *American Journal of Clinical Nutrition* 103: 1213–1223.

Lee, S., et al. 2017. Antibacterial activity of epigallocatechin-3-gallate (EGCG) and its synergism with β-lactam antibiotics sensitizing carbapenem-associated multidrug resistant clinical isolates of *Acinetobacter baumannii. Phytomedicine* 24: 49–55.

Liu, Q., et al. 2017. Antibacterial and antifungal activities of spices. *International Journal of Molecular Sciences,* June 16, online.

Maliakal, P., et al. 2011. Relevance of drug metabolizing enzyme activity modulation by tea polyphenols in the inhibition of esophageal tumorigenesis. *Medicinal Chemistry* 7: 480–487.

McKay, D. L., and Blumberg, J. B. 2006. A review of the bioactivity and potential health benefits of peppermint tea (*Mentha piperita* L.). *Phytotherapy Research* 20: 619–633.

Metzgar, C. J., et al. 2015. Facilitators and barriers to weight loss and weight loss maintenance: A qualitative exploration. *Journal of Human Nutrition and Dietetics* 28: 593–603.

Mohd Ali, N., et al. 2012. The promising future of chia, *Salvia hispanica* L. *Journal of Biomedicine and Biotechnology* 2012: 171956.

Morris, M. C., et al. 2006. Associations of vegetable and fruit consumption with age-related cognitive change. *Neurology* 24: 1370–1376.

Murphy, E. A., et al. 2010. Immune modulating effects of β-glucan. *Current Opinion in Clinical Nutrition and Metabolic Care* 13: 656–661.

Nabavi, S. F., et al. 2015. Anti-oxidative polyphenolic compounds of cocoa. *Current Pharmaceutical Biotechnology* 16: 891–901.

Ninfali, P., et al. 2017. C-glycosyl flavonoids from *Beta vulgaris cicla* and betalains from *Beta vulgaris rubra*: Antioxidant, anticancer and anti-inflammatory activities—a review. *Phytotherapy Research* 31: 871–884.

Panahi, Y., et al. 2016. *Chlorella vulgaris*: A multifunctional dietary supplement with diverse medicinal properties. *Current Pharmaceutical Design* 22: 164–173.

Popkin, B. M., and Nielsen, S. J. 2003. The sweetening of the world's diet. *Obesity Research* 11: 1325–1332.

Rastogi, S., et al. 2017. Spices: Therapeutic potential in cardiovascular health. *Current Pharmaceutical Design* 23: 989–998.

Rolls, B. J., et al. 2005. Increasing the volume of a food by incorporating air affects satiety in men. *American Journal of Clinical Nutrition* 72: 361–368.

Rolls, B. J., et al. 2005. Provision of foods differing in energy density affects long-term weight loss. *Obesity Research* 13:1052–1060.

Sadeghi, L., et al. 2016. Antioxidant effects of alfalfa can improve iron oxide nanoparticle damage: Invivo and invitro studies. *Regulatory Toxicology and Pharmacology* 81: 39–46.

Skrovankova, S., et al. 2012. Antioxidant activity and protecting health effects of common medicinal plants. *Advances in Food and Nutrition Research* 67: 75–139.

Suleria, H. A., et al. 2015. Onion: nature's protection against physiological threats. *Critical Reviews in Food Science and Nutrition* 55: 50–66.

Tang, D., et al. Pharmacokinetic properties and drug interactions of apigenin, a natural flavone. *Expert Opinion on Drug Metabolism and Toxicology* 13: 323–330.

Tang, Y., and Tsao, R. 2017. Phytochemicals in quinoa and amaranth grains and their antioxidant, anti-inflammatory, and potential health beneficial effects: A review. *Molecular Nutrition and Food Research*, April 18, online.

Tonstad, S., et al. 2014. A high-fibre bean-rich diet versus a low-carbohydrate diet for obesity. *Journal of Human Nutrition and Dietetics* 27 suppl. 2: 109–116.

Turner-McGrievy, G. M., et al. 2015. Comparative effectiveness of plant-based diets for weight loss: A randomized controlled trial of five different diets. *Nutrition* 31: 350–358.

Valdiva-Lopez, M. A., and Tecante, A. 2015. Chia (*Salvia hispanica*): A review of native Mexican seed and its nutritional and functional properties. *Advances in Food and Nutrition Research* 75: 53–75.

Van Hung, P. 2016. Phenolic compounds of cereals and their antioxidant capacity. *Critical Reviews in Food Science and Nutrition* 56: 25–35.

Xavier, A. A., and Perez-Galvez, A. 2016. Carotenoids as a source of antioxidants in the diet. *Sub-cellular Biochemistry* 79:359–375.

Yamaguchi, K. K., et al. 2015. Amazon açai: Chemistry and biological activities: A review. *Food Chemistry* 179: 137–151.

INDEX

Page numbers in **boldface** refer to recipes.

305

313

ABOUT THE AUTHOR

NIKKI SHARP is the author of the bestselling book *The 5-Day Real Food Detox*, creator of the hugely popular app *The 5-Day Detox*, health coach, yoga instructor, and vegan chef. What began as a passion to heal herself of an eating disorder has led her to helping hundreds of thousands around the world through her website and social media accounts.

Sharp has been featured in *Shape, Elle, Women's Fitness,* and *Men's Health,* and appeared on *Good Day LA, Access Hollywood Live,* and *Fox News.*

You can find her at home in Los Angeles creating a new recipe for her community, jumping on a plane to explore new cultures, or working out with friends, followed by a cheeky glass of wine.

nikkisharp.com
Instagram: @nikkisharp
Twitter: @NikkiRSharp
Facebook.com/nikkisharplimited